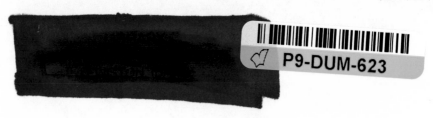
WITHDRAWN

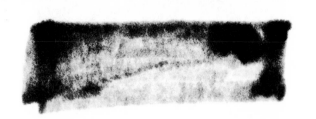

LONG-TERM CONDITIONS

SAGE has been part of the global academic community since 1965, supporting high quality research and learning that transforms society and our understanding of individuals, groups, and cultures. SAGE is the independent, innovative, natural home for authors, editors and societies who share our commitment and passion for the social sciences.

Find out more at: **www.sagepublications.com**

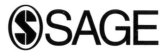

LONG-TERM CONDITIONS

CONDITIONS

Challenges in Health and Social Care

Edited by Cathy E. Lloyd and Tom Heller

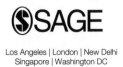

Los Angeles | London | New Delhi
Singapore | Washington DC

First published 2012

SAGE Publications Ltd
1 Oliver's Yard
55 City Road
London EC1Y 1SP

SAGE Publications Inc.
2455 Teller Road
Thousand Oaks, California 91320

SAGE Publications India Pvt Ltd
B 1/I 1 Mohan Cooperative Industrial Area
Mathura Road
New Delhi 110 044

SAGE Publications Asia-Pacific Pte Ltd
33 Pekin Street #02-01
Far East Square
Singapore 048763

Library of Congress Control Number: 2011927007

British Library Cataloguing in Publication data

A catalogue record for this book is available from the British Library

ISBN 978-0-85702-749-8
ISBN 978-0-85702-750-4 (pbk)

Typeset by C&M Digitals (P) Ltd, Chennai, India
Printed by MPG Books Group, Bodmin, Cornwall
Printed on paper from sustainable resources

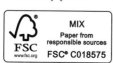

This book is dedicated to two wonderful women.

Elizabeth Simmons who bravely fought the debilitating consequences of her long-term conditions for many years and who was a dear friend and inspiration to Cathy Lloyd, and Elisabeth Hudson who was Tom Heller's mother-in-law and who was a role model for him in so many ways.

Table of Contents

Notes on the Editors and Contributors

Cathy E. Lloyd is an academic and researcher at the Open University, where she is a Senior Lecturer in the Faculty of Health and Social Care. She has been involved in teaching pre-registration nursing and courses in health care studies, where understanding the personal experience of long-term conditions is a central tenet. Her current research interests include the experience of co-morbid physical and mental illness, and in particular the impact of the ever increasing burden of diabetes and its psychological sequelae on both an individual as well as societal level. Recently the measurement of psychological wellbeing and the cultural applicability of existing tools to measure psychological distress in minority ethnic groups has been the focus of her funded research, which has led her to international collaborations with colleagues from the Dialogue on Diabetes and Depression (DDD) as well as from the European Association for the Study of Diabetes (EASD) Psychosocial Aspects of Diabetes Study Group.

Tom Heller has had parallel careers as a doctor and as an academic. Both paths have involved attempts to understand the issues and challenges that are faced by people with long-term conditions, their families and their formal and informal carers.

As a doctor he worked as a general practitioner in some of the most deprived areas of Sheffield where long-term illness is ever present and where it has become a major factor shaping the lives of many people living there. His work as an academic has centred around his appointment as a Senior Lecturer in Health at the Open University, Faculty of Health and Social Care, where for the last 25 years he has been involved in writing a wide range of health courses. His interests include mental health, complementary medicine and, of course, the way that long-term conditions affect the lives of people.

Katharine Barnard is a health psychologist at the University of Southampton. She has a longstanding research interest in the psychosocial issues associated with Type 1 diabetes in children, adolescents, adults and other family members. Through her research she has gained an in-depth understanding of the factors that contribute to quality of life and the impact of diabetes on daily living. The effect of diabetes, both medically and socially in terms of everyday coping, psychosocial impact and psychological burden, is a multifaceted and complex area and Dr Barnard's research to date has made significant advances in the unravelling of these complexities for individuals living with the condition.

Elaine Denny is Professor of Health Sociology at Birmingham City University. She has a background in hospital and community nursing and taught health sociology to students on health related courses for 20 years. Her research interests focus around women as recipients and providers of health care, and she has published work on women's experience of IVF, the experience of endometriosis, and on the occupation of nursing. Elaine has co-authored with Sarah Earle a health sociology text *Sociology for Nurses* the second edition of which was published in 2009. Also with Sarah Earle she has edited *The Sociology of Long-term Conditions*. Recent research includes a NHS Research for Patient Benefit funded collaborative study on endometriosis and cultural diversity aimed at improving services for minority ethnic women. She is also involved in exploring the patient perspective in a number of NHS NIHR funded clinical trials in collaboration with Birmingham Women's Hospital where she is an Honorary Research Associate.

Dr Sarah Earle is a medical sociologist with a special interest in reproductive and sexual health. She convened the British Sociological Association's Human Reproduction Study Group for nearly 14 years and her work spans across the field to include: pregnancy and childbirth, infant feeding, reproductive loss, commercial sex and sexual health services provision. She is currently Senior Lecturer in Health and Associate Dean for Research in the Faculty of Health and Social Care at The Open University. She is Sub-editor for Health and Social Sciences for the journal *Human Fertility*.

Andrew Gibson is a Research Fellow in Patient and Public Involvement (PPI) with the Peninsula Collaboration for Leadership in Applied Health Research and Care (PenCLAHRC). He has experience of evaluating user involvement in a number of contexts and he previously worked at the DH funded National Centre for Involvement at Warwick University. He also has experience of coordinating user involvement in research and teaching in the School of Health and Social Studies at Warwick University. He has responsibility for developing PPI within all the activities of PenCLAHRC.

His other research interests lie in the area of lay perspectives on health inequalities. His research in this area has drawn on the work of Bourdieu to explore the relationship between health, social status and social capital from the perspective of people living in a 'deprived' community.

Alistair Hewison is a Senior Lecturer in the School of Health and Population Sciences at the University of Birmingham. His professional background is in nursing, and he has experience as a staff nurse, charge nurse and manager in the NHS in Birmingham, Oxford and Warwickshire. Having undertaken a number of roles in Higher Education including Head of Nursing and Head of School, his current research and teaching activities are centred on the management and organisation of care. His main focus at the moment is a five year project examining service re-design in three acute NHS Trusts as part of the National Institute for Health Research funded Collaborations for Applied Health Research and Care programme in Birmingham and the Black Country (CLAHRC-BBC). He has written widely on health care management and policy issues in papers published in scholarly journals and chapters in edited collections.

Ruth Howard qualified as a Clinical Psychologist in 1996 and for many years worked in the area of cancer and palliative care, in clinical and academic roles. In 2000 she took up a post on the Clinical Psychology Training Course at the University of Birmingham and progressed to the role of Clinical Director in 2005, and more recently has moved into a Senior Academic Tutor on the course. She continues to work clinically in palliative care, and supervises research in this and other areas of health psychology, and over the last 4 years she has begun to develop research into the psychosocial impact of coeliac disease and its management. In 2008 she was awarded a grant by Coeliac UK to carry out a two-year study into the psychological and social implications of coeliac disease across the lifespan – the first study of its kind in the UK. This has led to the development of further research in this area and the establishment of the Coeliac Disease Research Steering Group at the University of Birmingham.

Mary Larkin is a Principal Lecturer in the Faculty of Health and Life Sciences, De Montfort University. She is also currently Programme Leader for the BA Health Studies and BSc Public and Community Health and has extensive experience of teaching on both undergraduate and postgraduate health and social care courses for a range of students, including health care professionals, in several higher education institutions. Her research interests are carers, carer empowerment adult social care, health and well-being, disability, and the third sector. She has carried out research at both national and international level as well as published widely about issues related to these research areas. Her publications also include several textbooks on health and social care.

Gary Law qualified as a Clinical Psychologist in 2000 and has worked clinically in the area of child psychology, child mental health and wellbeing for over 10 years. His current clinical post is in a Child and Adolescent Mental Health Service, where he leads the primary care service. In 2002 he joined the Clinical Psychology Training Course at the University of Birmingham and currently works as a Senior Academic Tutor and Lecturer. He contributes to the teaching and research supervision of undergraduate and postgraduate students. His research interests include child and family beliefs regarding chronic physical health and mental health, specifically the use of self-regulation theory to explore self-management and adjustment. Additional interests include the stigma of child mental health and predictors of help seeking.

Sara Mackian is a Senior Lecturer in Health and Wellbeing at The Open University. Formerly Lecturer in Health Geographies at the University of Manchester, the driving theme underpinning her research is a curiosity for how people, communities and organisations interact around issues of illness, health and wellbeing. This has led to a range of studies exploring ME, parenting, sexuality, spirituality and public health. A geographer by training, Sara has a particular interest in qualitative research methodologies, and has developed a method for 'mapping' data analysis, which she uses to visualize the worlds of experience revealed through her research, where the physical, socio-cultural, subjective and otherworldly intersect. She is author of *Everyday Spirituality: Social and Spatial Worlds of Enchantment* (Palgrave Macmillan).

Margo Milne is a researcher and a disabled service user living with a long-term condition. Her work includes both qualitative and quantitative research into the experiences of long-term conditions and attitudes towards end of life care, disability and physical illness. Her chapter focuses on the debates surrounding the overlap between disability, physical health and ill health, and the implications for receiving health and social care.

Stephen Pattison is an interdisciplinary scholar who presently serves as Professor of Religion, Ethics and Practice and HG Wood Professor of Theology at University of Birmingham where he is also head of the Department of Theology and Religion. An honorary professor in medical humanities in the School of Medicine and Health at Durham University, he also sits on the Ethics Committee of the Royal College of General Practitioners. Pattison is a former health care chaplain and consumer champion in the NHS. With interests in applied theology, management, visuality, values and ethics he is one of the co-editors and contributors to *Values in Professional Practice* (2004) and *Emerging Values in Health Care* (2010). Other recent and forthcoming publications include *Seeing Things: Deepening Relations with Visual Artefacts* (2007), *Face: Practical Theological Reflections* (2013), *Muslim Chaplaincy in England and Wales* (2013). Pattison was the founding co-ordinator of Think About Health (www.think abouthealth.com), an interdisciplinary reflective group dedicated to doing intellectual plumbing in the NHS.

Jane Petty conducted her PhD at the University of Birmingham with Professor Chris Oliver. The project explored self-injurious behaviour in children with severe intellectual disabilities and was completed in 2006. She then worked with Professor Oliver on a project looking at challenging behaviour in children and young adults with Angelman, Cri du Chat and Cornelia de Lange syndromes; genetic disorders associated with intellec-tual disability. In 2009, Jane moved into Health Psychology research, taking up a research fellow position with Drs Ruth Howard and Gary Law exploring psychosocial factors in coeliac disease. Her interest in Health Psychology continued to grow and she is currently working towards an MSc in Health Psychology via distance learning. Jane hopes to combine both her areas of expertise in future research and explore psychosocial issues associated with intellectual and physical disability, particularly from the parent/carer perspective.

Terry Pratchett needs no introduction; he is one of the most popular and prolific authors in the UK. He has established himself as a wonderfully resourceful and imaginative writer able to create whole new worlds for his cast of characters to inhabit … but he now has been given a diagnosis of early dementia. He has 'gone public' about his condition and written articles for the popular press and appeared on television programmes dis-cussing the condition in general and his prospects in particular. In his chapter Terry talks about some of his hopes and fears, as well as his early experiences of living with the condition.

Rachel Purtell is the Folk.us Director with day to day responsibility for Folk.us. This role ensures that service users, patients and carers are able to have a positive and meaningful impact on research, and the structures and processes that support research in health and social care. Rachel works with many people including people with learning difficulties, people who experienced mental distress, people with physical and/or sensory impairments, older people and people who are long-term users of the NHS. Rachel is a freelance trainer in Disability Equality Issues using a Social Model approach. She holds an MA in Disability Studies. She has a background in working for inclusive service user led organisations and delivers training. Rachel is disabled women, a disability activist and a service user.

Erica Richardson holds an honorary post in the European Centre on the Health of Societies in Transition (ECOHOST) at the London School of Hygiene and Tropical Medicine, while working for the European Observatory on Health Systems and Policies. Her research background is in Area Studies, analysing the development of public health policy and interventions in the field of substance abuse and HIV/AIDS prevention in the Russian Federation. Her current research focuses on health system reform in countries of the former Soviet Union but encompasses broader comparative work on health systems and policies in Europe. The aim of her work at the Observatory is to inform the comparative analysis of health systems and to raise awareness among policy-makers about international experience in health system reform. At LSHTM she teaches on the Masters in Public Health course.

Introduction

Cathy E. Lloyd and Tom Heller

This book has set itself a considerable challenge which is to explore the reality of the lives of people who develop long-term conditions and discuss some of the challenges for people who set out to care for them. The book takes a broad perspective which includes the worlds of both health and social care and contextualizes some of the diverse ways that people live with and experience these conditions.

Increasingly, people in developed countries can expect to live longer and this has important implications for long-term health and well-being. Many of the conditions that previously may have limited the length of a person's life can potentially be controlled and are no longer necessarily life threatening. Growing numbers of people experience more than one long-term condition, and this increasing complexity of need has important implications for both formal and informal types of health and social care provision.

The growing numbers of people in the UK living with long-term conditions has a serious impact on the way that resources within the NHS and the social care services are organized. There are also clear indications that there is a need throughout these services and in wider society for improved education and training for those living with long-term conditions, and also for carers and practitioners. Health and social care practitioners continue to be encouraged to work in partnership with people living with long-term conditions and with their carers. In order to reflect some of these dynamics the contributors to this book include people who identify themselves as having a long-term condition as well as authors drawn from a range of different academic disciplines. The authors have employed a range of research-related perspectives that reflect the need for multi-professional understanding of this complex subject area. Each chapter is based either on personal experience, or on empirical research and critical analysis of current policies and management of these conditions. The aim throughout has been to assist the reader in considering health and social care in context, bridging theory and practice, and challenging and inspiring current practice in health and social care.

The book is divided into three sections that reflect the different perspectives of a wide range of interested parties. This includes people who use services, carers, practitioners, managers and policy makers. At the same time each chapter uses empirical research to help the reader understand some of the realities associated with the provision of health and social care. The first section – Receiving Care – focuses on services users' experiences of health and social care, and includes the researched experiences of people who have a variety of different long-term conditions including ME, diabetes and Alzheimer's disease. The contributors to this section describe in detail service-users' perspectives on self-management of long-term conditions and the frequently experienced tensions between individual and health service priorities for care. The often unremitting, day to day need for self-care and the incorporation of the needs of illness into daily life is explored and discussed. A wide range of different perspectives and a variety of research methods underpin these chapters. For example in the first chapter Sir Terry Pratchett uses a very personal account that could be described as an auto-ethnographic approach to describe his experience of the early stages of Alzheimer's disease. Subsequent chapters utilize a wide variety of other types of research data, both qualitative and quantitative.

The second section of this book – Working with People with Long-term Conditions – focuses on some of the ways that practitioners and service users may be able to work together in a range of settings in order to improve the lives of people with a variety of long-term conditions. The dilemmas experienced by GPs and other health care workers when faced with difficult decisions in the provision of care are considered. In addition some of the ways that research, and especially service user involvement in research, can inform practice are outlined. This section also includes a consideration of some of the different approaches to disability within the field of health and social care, and the implications for practitioners working with disabled people. Integral to these contemporary issues are debates around partnerships in care, empowering practice, inter-professional working and effective communication in health and social care.

The final section of this book – Delivering Health and Social Care for People with Long-term Conditions – focuses on policy, organizations, and ways in which the complex needs of individuals with long-term conditions are managed across the boundaries of health and social care. The chapters in this section have been designed to give the reader an up-to-date understanding of some of the policy-related debates concerning care provision for people with long-term conditions. Current concerns around the growing number of people living with long-term conditions and the quality and increasing complexity of care provision are explored. The daunting organizational constraints in delivering care are considered and the implications for future practice discussed. Some of the complex ethical issues involved in delivering care for people with long-term conditions as well as the importance of making a clinical diagnosis and the role of carers in supporting this group of people are also explored.

This book gives the reader a chance to gain an in-depth understanding of the experience of long-term ill-health from a range of perspectives. Together the contributors have provided an opportunity to critically reflect on both the boundaries between health and social care provision, and the importance of evidence in understanding health and ill-health, and learn about current policy drives towards improved inter-professional working. We hope the collection will help people who are service users as well as health and social care practitioners move towards a greater under-standing of integrated care, the complexity of needs, and multi-professional working. The various chapters also point to key areas for future research.

This book is the result of many different people's hard work and we would like to take this opportunity to thank them all. In particular a vote of thanks goes to all our colleagues who contributed to this book, to our Editorial Assistant at Sage, Emma Milman, and to Billy Simmons who made many suggestions for the book cover.

Cathy E. Lloyd, PhD
Open University
Faculty of Health and Social Care

Tom Heller, MB, BS
Open University
Faculty of Health and Social Care

SECTION ONE

RECEIVING CARE

Introduction

Cathy E. Lloyd

People currently living in developed countries can expect to live longer than their predecessors, but at the same time are faced with the likelihood that they will be diagnosed with one or more long-term conditions during their extended lifetime. This has implications for formal and informal health and social care services in these countries because people will increasingly need more care for longer periods of time. Previous research has traditionally been seen from the perspective of health care professionals and has often focused on biomedical cures for disease rather than on ways that people may be able to cope with conditions that are not curable, only manageable. More recently there has been a shift towards research that focuses on managing long-term conditions in order to maintain an acceptable quality of life. This re-focus emphasizes each individual's ability to self-manage their own health and illness. The first section of this book brings together some of this novel research and focuses on personal experiences of long-term conditions and the health and social care that has been received.

The first contribution to this section is entitled 'Living with Early Dementia' from Sir Terry Pratchett. Sir Terry is one of the most popular and prolific authors in the UK. He has established himself as a wonderfully resourceful and imaginative writer able to create whole new worlds for his cast of characters to inhabit – but he now has been given a diagnosis of early dementia. He has 'gone public' about his condition and written articles for the popular press and appeared on television programmes discussing the condition in general and his prospects in particular. In this chapter he talks about some of his hopes and fears, as well as his early experiences of living with the condition.

The following chapters are also from contributors who have experience of particular long-term conditions as well as having conducted research in the field. Margo Milne takes an auto-ethnographic approach in her chapter, 'Disability and Illness: The Perspectives of People Living with a Long-term Condition', and combines her own personal experience of multiple sclerosis (MS) with her empirical research into this long-term condition. She asks the question: 'Is it a physical problem or a disability?' and debates issues surrounding the overlap between disability, physical health and ill-health, and the implications for receiving health and social care. This chapter contains a consideration of the appropriateness of different methodological approaches to researching these sensitive issues and discusses ways of ensuring that the voices of people living with long-term conditions are heard.

The experience of having a long-term physical condition can be made more complex when other health problems occur at the same time. Having more than one long-term condition, often called 'co-morbidity', is the subject of the next chapter by Katharine Barnard and Cathy E. Lloyd. Both these authors have been researching in the field of diabetes and mental health for a number of years and in their chapter they review some of that research. The chapter, 'Experiencing Depression and Diabetes', focuses on the experience of having diabetes as well as depression. People with diabetes have to grapple with the heavy, constant burden of having to look after their own condition and it is no wonder that they run a greatly increased risk of developing mental health problems, especially depression. The combination of physical and mental health difficulties often leads to serious challenges for the provision of appropriate care. This chapter reviews some of the empirical evidence of increased rates of depression in people with this long-term condition. More recent research on the impact of self-management on feelings of diabetes distress or 'burnout' is also described and discussed. The difficulties for health workers of identifying whether a person with diabetes is feeling depressed, or whether they have become distressed about the management of their diabetes, are also debated.

The chapter entitled, 'Experiencing and Managing Medically Unexplained Conditions: The Case of Chronic Pelvic Pain in Women', has been contributed by Elaine Denny. She explores the impact of being assigned the label of 'unexplained' for women experiencing pelvic pain. This chapter focuses on the concept of 'expert knowledge' and discusses whose knowledge should be considered to be more 'legitimate'. Diagnosis has become an integral element of biomedicine that provides legitimation of symptoms and confers credibility on people who are living the reality of those unexplained symptoms. This is important because without a recognized diagnosis entitlement to services and treatment is open to question. However for many doctors Chronic Pelvic Pain remains a controversial and contested condition. This adds another level of complexity that women with this condition have to negotiate in their passage through the formal health care system.

The final chapter in this section of the book is written by Sara Mackian who is an academic, a researcher, and also a service user with ME. She takes an auto-ethnographic approach in her chapter, 'Me and ME: Therapeutic Landscapes in an Unfamiliar World'. This chapter is underpinned by her empirical research alongside other people with ME. She explores how this condition, for which biomedicine can define no clear cause and currently offers no effective treatment, can leave the individual beyond the safety net of formal service provision. This means that many people find themselves feeling isolated and have to negotiate a 'new normality' which works for them and their condition. ME has serious implications for physical engagement with the world and the condition often leaves people shut off and unable to interact. However, Sara's research investigates some of the creative ways in which people with ME may be able to fashion new subjective, social or spiritual worlds to help them cope with their experiences.

This section of the book brings together research into the way that people living with long-term conditions view the management of their own situation and their health concerns. Much of the empirical evidence cited in these chapters comes from in-depth qualitative research, demonstrating the importance of these methods in understanding individuals' experiences of long-term conditions.

1

Living with Early Dementia

Sir Terry Pratchett

> **Overview**
>
> - Clapham Junction days
> - Obtaining a diagnosis of early Alzheimer's
> - Undeniable signs
> - Disease of knowledge

People who have dementia in this country are not heard. I'm fortunate; I can be heard. Regrettably, it's amazing how people listen if you stand up in public and give away $1million for research into the disease, as I have done. Why did I do it? I regarded finding I had a form of Alzheimer's as an insult and decided to do my best to marshall any kind of forces I could against this wretched disease.

I have posterior cortical atrophy or PCA. They say, rather ingenuously, that if you have Alzheimer's it's the best form of Alzheimer's to have. This is a moot point, but what it does do, while gradually robbing you of memory, visual acuity and other things you didn't know you had until you miss them, is leave you more or less as fluent and coherent as you always have been.

I spoke to a fellow sufferer recently (or as I prefer to say, 'a person who is thoroughly annoyed with the fact they have dementia') who talked in the tones of a university lecturer and in every respect was quite capable of taking part in an animated conversation. Nevertheless, he could not see the teacup in front of him. His eyes knew that the cup was there; his brain was not passing along the information. This disease slips you away a little bit at a time and lets you watch it happen.

This is a slightly edited version of an article first published in the *Daily Mail*.

When I look back now, I suspect there may be some truth in the speculation that dementia (of which Alzheimer's is the most common form) may be present in the body for quite some time before it can be diagnosed. For me, things came to a head in the late summer of 2007. My typing had been getting progressively worse and my spelling had become erratic. I grew to recognize what I came to call Clapham Junction days when the demands of the office grew too much to deal with.

I was initially diagnosed not with Alzheimer's but with an ischemic change, a simple loss of brain cells due to normal ageing. That satisfied me until the next Clapham Junction day. I went back to my GP and said I knew there was something more going on. Fortunately, she knew well enough not to bother with the frankly pathetic MMSE test (the 30-point questionnaire used to determine brain function) and sent me to Addenbrooke's Hospital in Cambridge, where, after examination of my MRI scan and an afternoon of complex tests, I was diagnosed with PCA, an uncommon variant of dementia, which had escaped the eagle eye of the original diagnostician.

When in *Paradise Lost* Milton's Satan stood in the pit of hell and raged at heaven, he was merely a trifle miffed compared to how I felt that day. I felt totally alone, with the world receding from me in every direction and you could have used my anger to weld steel. Only my family and the fact I had fans in the medical profession, who gave me useful advice, got me through that moment. I feel very sorry for, and angry on behalf of, the people who don't have the easy ride I had.

It is astonishing how long it takes some people to get diagnosed (I know because they write to me). I cannot help but wonder if this is because doctors are sometimes reluctant to give the patient the stigma of dementia since there is no cure.

I was extremely fortunate in my GP. I think she was amazed to find that of the two specialists in my area, one had no experience of PCA and therefore did not feel he could help me and the other would only take on patients over 65 – at 59 I was clearly too young to have Alzheimer's.

I remember on that day of rage thinking that if I'd been diagnosed with cancer of any kind, at least there would have opened in front of me a trodden path. There would have been specialists, examinations; there would be in short, some machinery in place. I was not in the mood for a response that said, more or less, 'go away and come back in six years'.

My wife said: 'Thank goodness it isn't a brain tumour', but all I could think then was: 'I know three people who have got better after a brain tumour. I haven't heard of anyone who's got better from Alzheimer's'.

It was my typing and spelling that convinced me the diagnosis was right. They had gone haywire. Other problems I put down to my looming 60th birthday. I thought no one else had noticed the fumbling with seat belts and the several attempts to get clothing on properly, but my wife and PA were worrying. We still have the occasional Clapham Junction day, now understood and dealt with.

I have written 47 novels in the past 25 years, but now I have to check the spelling of even quite simple words – they just blank on me at random. I would not dare to write this without the once despised checker, and you would have your work cut out to read it, believe me. On the other hand – and this is very typical of PCA – when the kind lady who periodically checks me out asked me to name as many animals as I can, I started with the rock hyrax, the nearest living relative to the elephant, and thylacine – the probably extinct Tasmanian marsupial wolf. That's the gift or the curse of our little variant. We have problems handling the physical world but can come pretty close to talking our way out of it so you don't notice. We might have our shirts done up wrong, but might be able to convince you it's a new style.

I felt that all I had was a voice, and I should make it heard. It never occurred to me not to use it. I went on the net and told, well, everyone. I wish I could say it was an act of bravery. It wasn't and I find that suggestion very nearly obscene. How brave is it to say you have a disease that does not hint of a dissolute youth, riotous living or even terrible eating habits? Anyone can contract dementia; and every day and with a growing momentum, anybody does.

It occurred to me that at one point it was like I had two diseases – one was Alzheimer's and the other was knowing I had Alzheimer's. There were times when I thought I'd have been much happier not knowing, just accepting that I'd lost brain cells and one day they'd probably grow back or whatever. It is better to know, though, and better for it to be known, because it has got people talking, which I rather think was what I had in mind. The $1 million I pledged to the Alzheimer's Research Trust was just to make them talk louder for a while.

It is a strange life when you 'come out'. People get embarrassed, lower their voices, get lost for words. Fifty per cent of Britons think there is a stigma surrounding dementia but only 25% think there is still a stigma associated with cancer. It seems that when you have cancer you are a brave battler against the disease, but when you have Alzheimer's you are an old fart. That's how people see you. It makes you feel quite alone. It seems to me there's hardly one family in this country that is not touched by the disease somehow. But people don't talk about it because it is so frightening. I swear that people think that if they say the word they're summoning the demon. It used to be the same with cancer.

Journalists, on the other hand – I appreciate that other people living with the disease don't get so much of this – find it hard to talk to me about anything else, and it dominates every interview: Yes, I said I had PCA ten months ago, yes, I still have it, yes, I wish I didn't, no, there is no cure.

I can't really object to all this, but it is strange that a disease that attracts so much attention, awe, fear and superstition is so underfunded in treatment and research. We don't know what causes it, and as far as we know the only way to be sure of not developing it is to die young. Regular exercise and eating sensibly are a good idea, but they don't come with any guarantees. There is no cure. Researchers are talking about the possibility of a whole palette of treatments or regimes to help those people with dementia to live active and satisfying lives, with the disease kept in reasonably permanent check in very much the same way as treatments now exist for HIV. Not so much a cure therefore as – we hope – a permanent reprieve. We hope it will come quickly, and be affordable.

When my father was in his terminal year, I discussed death with him. I recall very clearly his relief that the cancer that was taking him was at least allowing him 'all his marbles'. Dementia in its varied forms is not like cancer. Dad saw the cancer in his pancreas as an invader. But Alzheimer's is me unwinding, losing trust in myself, a butt of my own jokes and on bad days capable of playing hunt the slipper by myself and losing.

You can't battle it, you can't be a plucky 'survivor'. It just steals you from yourself. And I'm 60; that's supposed to be the new 40. The baby boomers are getting older, and will stay older for longer. And they will run right into the dementia firing range. How will a society cope? Especially a society that can't so readily rely on those stable family relationships that traditionally provided the backbone of care?

What is needed is will and determination. The first step is to talk openly about dementia because it's a fact, well enshrined in folklore, that if we are to kill the demon then first we have to say its name. Once we have recognized the demon, without secrecy or shame, we can find its weaknesses. Regrettably one of the best swords for killing demons like this is made of gold – lots of gold. These days we call it funding. I believe the D-day battle on Alzheimer's will be engaged shortly and a lot of things I've heard from experts, not always formally, strengthen that belief. It's a physical disease, not some mystic curse; therefore it will fall to a physical cure. There's time to kill the demon before it grows.

Summary

This is a personal account by an acclaimed and accomplished author who, at the time of writing, had just been diagnosed with Alzheimer's disease.

We are proud that he has given us permission to use his writing as the first chapter in our collection about long-term conditions. This chapter emphasizes the importance of listening to the people who have long-term conditions. What they have to say is always important, but it may not be what health and social care professionals were expecting.

Further reading

Alzheimer's Society website: http://alzheimers.org.uk/

Bayley, J. (1998) *Iris: A Memoir of Iris Murdoch*. London: Duckworth.

Beaumont, H. (2009) *Loosing Clive to Younger Onset Dementia: One Family's Story*. London: Jessica Kingsley.

Brooker, D. (2007) *Person-centred Dementia Care: Making Services Better*. London: Jessica Kingsley.

Bryden, C. (2005) *Dancing with Dementia: My Story of Living Positively with Dementia*. London: Jessica Kingsley.

Cox, S. and Keady, J. (1999) *Younger People with Dementia: Planning, Practice and Development*. London: Jessica Kingsley

Downs, M. and Bowers, B. (2008) *Excellence in Dementia Care: Research into Practice*. Milton Keynes: Open University Press.

Hughes, J. and Baldwin, C. (2006) *Ethical Issues in Dementia Care: Making Difficult Decisions*. London: Jessica Kingsley.

Kitwood, T. (1997) *Dementia Reconsidered: The Person Comes First*. Buckingham: Oxford University Press.

Perrin, T., May, H. and Anderson, E. (2008) *Wellbeing in Dementia*. Edinburgh: Elsevier.

2

Disability and Illness: The Perspectives of People Living with a Long-term Condition

Margo Milne with Mary Larkin and Cathy E. Lloyd

Overview

- Ways of looking at impairment, disability and illness
- Why a long-term condition can be perceived as both an illness and a disability
- The invisibility of disabilities
- Disability and the self
- Disability as both sickness and health

Demographic changes are certain to mean that there will continue to be an increase in the total number of people with long-term conditions and disabilities in the UK (Office for National Statistics, 2009; Shakespeare and Watson, 2002). Translated into actual numbers, the Office for Disability Issues (2008) estimated that there were nearly 10 million disabled adults in the UK, with around 5 million of these people being over state pension age. The definition of disability used in the collection of these figures was 'having a longstanding illness, disability or infirmity, and having a significant difficulty with day-to-day activities'. This definition implies a link or overlap between illness and disability, which can be further understood through examining the experiences of people with certain long-term conditions. Using research reports of people with Multiple Sclerosis (MS) as well as my own experience of this condition, this chapter will explore how these blurred boundaries can lead to a range of challenging experiences when receiving health and social care. The box, 'Margo's story' puts you in the picture with regards my own experience of having a long-term condition and disability:

Margo's story

For around 15 years, I made repeated visits to a series of general practitioners, complaining of severe fatigue. On each occasion, I was met with platitudes like 'But everyone gets tired'. It seemed impossible to explain that this wasn't normal tiredness – I knew what that felt like and this wasn't it! Sometimes I was offered anti-depressants, but with a previous history of major depression, I knew that was not the problem at that time.

It was only in 2003, when my health broke down completely, that my GP began to do investigations. I began to have severe dizziness and pass out, my fatigue was now overwhelming, and within a few months I needed a wheelchair to go more than a hundred yards.

The investigations took nearly two years. The uncertainty during this period only added to the stress of having a major and progressive condition. I was imagining myself to have every condition from Motor Neurone Disease to a brain tumour. Finally, in March 2005, I was diagnosed as having Multiple Sclerosis (MS), a condition that is made worse by stress. As I was able to identify relapse-like episodes dating back at least 15 years, the neurologist diagnosed me immediately as having the secondary progressive type. I had an illness (or rather a long-term condition) and I was also disabled.

By this time, I was having to use a power wheelchair whenever I left home, and was being visited by carers every morning. While using a wheelchair undoubtedly gives me more independence physically, I do feel frustrated by inaccessible premises and events. I am also made angry by insensitive and thoughtless comments from those who presumably have no experience of disability.

I get frustrated when I 'fall into the gaps' of care: for instance when there is a break in a prescription between the initial supply from a hospital doctor and the repeat supply from my GP. It is frustrating, too, when health care professionals will not listen to my knowledge of how my condition affects me, and try to apply a one-size-fits-all remedy. A physiotherapist refused to believe that I was having cognitive (thinking) problems 'because you're studying for a PhD'. This was annoying beyond belief.

The 'invisible' symptoms of my disability remain the most difficult for others to understand. Lack of mobility is easy to comprehend: fatigue and pain not so. As subjective experiences, they are hard to communicate, and as everyday words, everyone has their own definition and experience of them. I have a number of

(Continued)

ongoing symptoms or 'illnesses', such as frequent infections, but fatigue is my biggest enemy. I have used the Spoon Theory (Miserandino, 2010), to explain severe fatigue to people, and know many others who have done the same. My social life now mainly revolves around other people with MS and a few others who are able to understand that I may need to cancel things at very short notice if I have a 'bad day'.

I don't know what the future holds. All I know is that my condition will progress: I don't know how fast, or how far. This uncertainty is one of the hallmarks of MS, and one of the most difficult things to deal with.

My experiences, briefly outlined above, specifically highlighted the lack of a clear distinction between illness and a disability, as well as the invisibility of disability, the juxtaposition of health and illness in disability and the role of professional attitudes in the experience of disability. These were also constant themes in my research with people with MS, discussed here in relation to recent literature and highlighting the implications for health and social care practice.

Illness or disability?

The *International Classification of Functioning, Disability and Health*, known more commonly as ICF (WHO, 2002), is an official classification of health and health-related domains. These domains are classified by means of two lists: a list of body functions and structure, and a list of domains of activity and participation. Since an individual's functioning and disability occurs in a context, the ICF also includes a list of environmental factors. In this classification body functions are defined in a very narrow, medicalized way, but domains of activity include a wide range of self-care, social, spiritual and political activities. Environmental factors include physical and social barriers, support and relationships, attitudes, and policies. In spite of the inclusion of these factors, this classification is usually considered to represent one of the *medical models of disability*.

From the late 1960s onwards, many disabled people have campaigned for more of a role for themselves when disability is defined. For example in 1976 the Union of the Physically Impaired Against Segregation (UPIAS) proposed this definition for the *social model of disability*:

In our view, it is society which disables physically impaired people. Disability is something imposed on top of our impairment by the way we are unnecessarily isolated and excluded from full participation in society. Disabled people are therefore an oppressed group in society.

Thus we define impairment as lacking part or all of a limb, organ or mechanism of the body; and disability as the disadvantage or restriction of activity caused by a contemporary social organisation which takes no or little account of people who have physical impairments and thus excludes them from participation in the mainstream of social activities. Physical impairment is therefore a particular form of social oppression. (UPIAS, 1976: 14)

Within this definition, disability becomes oppression placed by society on people with impairments. Impairment is a prerequisite of disability (Finkelstein, 2001), but disability does not necessarily follow from impairment. In this chapter, however, I will continue to use the term 'disability' in its everyday sense, to include physical impairments.

The distinction between impairment and disability is important to many disabled people because it removes the 'blame' for their oppressed position in society. Many of the structures of bureaucracy seem designed to make the disabled person aware of how they fail to meet the 'norm'. For example, claimants for Disability Living Allowance, which aims to provide finance for people with mobility and personal care needs, have to describe themselves using negative terminology, as an incapable person rather than in positive terms (Reeve, 2002). It is my contention here that when health care professionals are working with people with disabilities and long-term conditions, using the social model and emphasizing positive aspects of their lives is not just a theoretical position, but a vital part of understanding.

Illness is what is perceived by the person living with it, as opposed to disease, which is a condition diagnosed and treated by doctors (Eisenberg, 1977). Many disabilities are disabilities only – the individuals concerned remain in good health, with no 'illness' present. One participant in my research, who has cerebral palsy, is offended if anyone refers to him as 'ill', as he does not consider himself to be so. In other situations, an individual may be considered to be 'ill' but not 'disabled', for instance by asymptomatic conditions such as the early stages of type 2 diabetes.

Some conditions may lead to both illness and disability, as in the case of MS. Multiple sclerosis is a debilitating condition in which the body's own immune system begins to destroy the protective sheath covering some of the nerves. This interferes with communication between the brain and the rest of the body. Ultimately, this may result in damage to the nerves themselves. Multiple sclerosis can occur at any age, but is most commonly diagnosed between the ages of 20 and 40. Women are about twice as likely to develop it as men. White people, particularly those of Northern European descent, are at highest risk of developing multiple sclerosis; people of Asian,

African and Native American descent are at lowest risk (Mayo Clinic Staff, 2009).

The symptoms of MS can vary widely and can be perceived as either part of the illness itself or can lead to disability, or both, depending on the amount and location of damage. The symptoms may include numbness or weakness in one or more limbs, partial or complete loss of vision, double vision or blurring of vision, tingling or pain, tremor, or dizziness (Mayo Clinic Staff, 2009). Extreme fatigue is probably the most common symptom of multiple sclerosis (Bakshi, 2003; Multiple Sclerosis Encyclopaedia, 2008; Kos et al., 2008; Smith and Hale, 2007). Along with a high prevalence of depression (Chwastiak et al., 2002; Patten et al., 2003; Siegert and Abernethy, 2005) and general malaise, this often leads to MS being perceived by those with it as an illness as much as a disability. People with multiple sclerosis often have very frequent contact with health care professionals for such things as catheter and bowel care or treatment of infections (Hennessey et al., 1999), reinforcing the perception of MS as an illness as well as a disability.

My own experience gives a good example of MS as both an illness and disability; as I mention in my story above, I have a number of ongoing symptoms or 'illnesses' which force me into frequent contact with health practitioners, underlining the blurred boundaries between illness and being a disabled person with a long-term condition. Having multiple long-term conditions almost always means that health and social care is required from a range of specialties. Furthermore individuals with one long-term condition often have to visit a number of different specialists: I myself am currently under the care of a neurologist, an MS specialist nurse, a continence specialist nurse, a urologist, a gastroenterologist, wheelchair services, a physiotherapist and an occupational therapist, as well of course as my GP and practice nurse. I also have daily visits from carers. This can lead to fragmentation of care and frequently to frustration due to lack of co-ordination between the different services involved.

Many people with MS have noticeable decrements in health-related quality of life and research has indicated that individuals with more than one long-term condition may experience an even poorer quality of life (Sprangers et al., 2000). The effect of disability on daily living is thought to be greater in MS than in many other long-term conditions (Devins et al., 1993). Other common features include anxiety, depression, and cognitive impairment (Feinstein, 2004; Patti, 2009). There is increasing recognition that these issues form a vital component of people's health-related quality of life, distinct from physical disability alone (Mitchell et al., 2005). However not all people with MS have both illness and disability; some may have mobility problems, for instance, without any of the 'illness' symptoms such as fatigue and pain. Many others, particularly in the early stages, have only 'illness' symptoms and no obvious disability. People can move between categories at different stages of their condition.

The invisibility of disability

Many symptoms of multiple sclerosis are invisible, and can be hard for others to appreciate and accept. There can be a perception that disabilities have to be visible to be 'taken seriously' (Stone, 2005). I have myself encountered professional care staff who held (and expressed) the opinion that I am not 'really' disabled because I am able to walk short distances – ignoring the reality of the pain and fatigue this causes me. It is particularly hard for people with MS to explain to others the all-pervading, crippling fatigue that many of us experience. It is often easiest to use an analogy, such as *The Spoon Theory*, in which Christine Miserandino, an American woman with a long-term condition called 'lupus', uses a bundle of teaspoons to describe the restrictions of long-term conditions (Miserandino, 2010).

Miserandino wanted to convey how people with a long-term condition often have a limited amount of energy with which to tackle everyday life. Each expenditure of energy, or each activity undertaken, leads to less available energy for any subsequent activities. She likened each energy expenditure to a spoon; with a limited number of spoons in the bundle it is important to be aware of the effects of each activity. One could 'borrow' a spoon from the next day's supply but that simply meant you would have less to use tomorrow and what if that day you become ill; '…you do not want to run low on spoons, because you never know when you will truly need them' (Miserandino, 2010).

I am aware anecdotally of many people with MS who have used *The Spoon Theory* to explain MS fatigue to family and friends, with some success. It could also increase understanding during consultations, and underlines the importance of health and social care practitioners listening to service users' own explanations of their symptoms and experiences. Miserandino's use of spoons as a metaphor for energy also mirrors other uses of metaphor in writings on health, most memorably perhaps by the American literary theorist Susan Sontag, who drew out the similarities between public perspectives on cancer and tuberculosis, and how both had become associated with particular psychological traits (Sontag, 1978).

Disability and the self

Research indicates that people with visible disabilities are likely to report poorer adjustment and self-concept than people with invisible disabilities:

for instance Goldberg found that children with a visible disability (facial burns) had lower levels of adjustment than children with an invisible disability (heart disease) (Goldberg, 1974). Tam and colleagues, working with Hong Kong Chinese adults, found that those with visible disabilities scored significantly lower in self-concept than did either the non-disabled control group or the group with disabilities that were not visible (Tam et al., 2003). However in the case of multiple sclerosis, it seems that invisible, illness-related symptoms such as pain and depression may cause more distress than visible ones such as problems with mobility (White et al., 2008). This may be because of the unpredictability of MS, and the subsequent difficulties in planning day to day life (Charmaz, 1991). As a female participant in my research said: 'My condition is different day to day, week to week'.

Some people with long-term conditions may hold a specific ideology about living with such conditions, with residuals, for instance, of the Protestant work ethic. These ideologies are predicated on values of hard work, independence and individual responsibility. Maintaining a 'normal' life or returning to one as soon as possible becomes a symbol of a valued self. People living with long-term conditions may view physical dependency as negative, and often blame themselves for it (Charmaz, 1983). In my own research three women I interviewed discussed their fear of dependency in the following ways:

> 'Becoming totally dependent with a terminal illness is something I am dreading.'
>
> 'I could not bear to live a completely dependent life.'
>
> 'I worry about becoming incapable of looking after myself.'

However another woman with MS took a more critical approach:

> 'I do question the fear of dependency. Is this a fear of the standard of care, and the loss of dignity and respect? – if so, this needs to be addressed in our society.'

Susan Wendell, an academic with myalgic encephalitis/chronic fatigue and immune dysfunction syndrome (ME/CFIDS), clearly resents every relapse:

> At the beginning of a relapse, I cannot help noticing that I am more easily exhausted every day, but I still resist giving in to being sick. The increasing fatigue feels like a progressive humiliation of my will and ego as it forces me to cancel my plans and retreat to my bed. (Wendell, 2008: 209)

I can empathize with Wendell: as someone with MS, I am regularly told to 'listen to my body', to rest when I need to. This makes it no easier to cancel social activities at the last minute or put off important deadlines. It is important for health care practitioners to *listen* to their clients, for instance if they say they have important commitments that cannot be put off. As my own story shows, health care practitioners can make assumptions about the effects of disability or illness that may or may not be true in terms of individual experience.

Having a serious long-term illness threatens the integrity of the self by disturbing previous assumptions about the relation between the body and the self. It undermines the self and identity (Charmaz, 1995), and can leave the individual with an over-riding stigmatized identity (Goffman, 1963). With progressive conditions, this process is continually repeated as the individual tries to re-establish the integrity of the self. It may be, therefore, that people with MS are more likely to report distress from invisible symptoms than visible ones, in contrast to the other research reported above, because MS causes more 'illness' symptoms than the other conditions researched. With its uncertain, variably progressive course, it forces the individual through an iterative process of self-definition.

Disability as both sickness and health

Strict dichotomous classifications such as well/unwell or health/illness are often inappropriate, especially when it comes to long-term conditions. Aaron Antonovsky, an Israeli American sociologist who worked on the relationship between stress, health and healing, proposed a continuum model, which sees each of us at any given point of time somewhere along a 'health-ease-dis-ease' continuum. This moves away both from medicine's traditional focus on those in need of a cure, and from health promotion's tendency to focus on avoiding risk factors for disease (Antonovsky, 1996). Individuals with long-term conditions may place themselves at a range of different points on this continuum, however many people with MS find themselves towards the 'dis-ease' end of the continuum, as did the three participants in my research who described their physical symptoms of MS in the following terms:

'My MS makes me feel fatigued. As soon as I wake up I am tired.'

'It [...] produces pain all the time. I guess that is always part of your thoughts so it will affect your life in everything you do.'

'Any physical activity especially tires me quickly and causes pain.'

Other research participants with MS spoke in terms of their condition 'getting worse' over time and the implications of this for their future health and well-being. As one woman said,

'I worry about becoming incapable of looking after myself which I can barely do now and need lots of help.'

However another research participant, who was born with a progressive condition, challenged these ideas of the worsening of her condition:

'Worse, that's an interesting concept, isn't it? Because I mean, I use terms like that, and I just say it, and I think what have I just said? I mean I have a progressive condition and my body will change, I do talk occasionally about getting worse, but actually I don't … if I, if I think about it properly I don't think about it as getting worse, I think about it as my physical state changing … and yet, society's terminology has become so inside me that you just trot it out.'

People such as those who took part in my research may move back and forwards along Antonovsky's continuum, depending on the stage of their condition, whether or not they are having a relapse, and whether they are having a good or bad day. An important message for health and social care practitioners is the need to remember that clients will not necessarily always be experiencing the same symptoms of either illness or disability.

Despite the often negative experiences of having a long-term condition, many individuals consider themselves to be in good health, despite disease. This dimension of health was one of nine identified by Mildred Blaxter (1990), one of the most influential writers in the health and social care field. Her research findings have been mirrored in government surveys. For example in one report, of all men and women over 65 in the UK reporting a long-term illness that limits their daily activities, just over 10% considered themselves to be in good health and another 45% reported themselves as being in fairly good health (OPCS, 2005).

Summary

This chapter has considered the relationship between the terms 'illness' and 'disability', and has used the experiences of people with MS, including my own, to illustrate how illness and disability may sometimes be at odds with each other but may at other times overlap or reinforce one another. My own experiences and those of the people I have met through my research have often been similar. MS can be perceived or experienced as both an illness and a disability and this can depend on where the individual with the condition is at any point in time on the health–dis-ease continuum. Many disabilities are 'invisible', however regardless of the visibility of long-term conditions they may still impact on the individual's sense of self or self-worth. The impact of long-term conditions such as MS can be difficult for those without the disease to appreciate, particularly at times of invisibility or apparent health/absence of sickness. This has important implications for the delivery of health and social care, especially given these changes in health status and the need for service-user focused care.

Further reading

Antonovsky, A. (1996) 'The salutogenic model as a theory to guide health promotion', *Health Promotion International*, 11: 11–18.

Charmaz, K. (1983) 'Loss of self: a fundamental form of suffering in the chronically ill', *Sociology of Health & Illness*, 5: 168–95.

Miserandino, C. (2010) *The Spoon Theory by Christine Miserandino: But You Don't Look Sick?* [Online]. Available at http://www.butyoudontlooksick.com/articles/written-by-christine/the-spoon-theory-written-by-christine-miserandino/

MS Society website: www.mssociety.org.uk

Sontag, S. (1978) *Illness as Metaphor*. London: Penguin.

References

Antonovsky, A. (1996) 'The salutogenic model as a theory to guide health promotion', *Health Promotion International*, 11: 11–18.

Bakshi, R. (2003) 'Fatigue associated with multiple sclerosis: Diagnosis, impact and management', *Multiple Sclerosis*, 9: 219–27.

Blaxter, M. (1990) *Health and Lifestyles*. London: Routledge.

Charmaz, K. (1983) 'Loss of self: A fundamental form of suffering in the chronically ill', *Sociology of Health & Illness*, 5: 168–95.

Charmaz, K. (1991) *Good Days, Bad Days: The Self in Chronic Illness and Time*. New Brunswick: Rutgers University Press.

Charmaz, K. (1995) 'The body, identity and self: Adapting to impairment', *Sociological Quarterly*, 36: 657–80.

Chwastiak, L., Ehde, D.M., Gibbons, L.E., Sullivan, M., Bowen, J.D. and Kraft, G.H. (2002) 'Depressive symptoms and severity of illness in multiple sclerosis: Epidemiologic study of a large community sample', *American Journal of Psychiatry*, 159: 1862–8.

Devins, G., Edworthy, S., Seland, T., Klein, G., Paul, I. and Mandin, H. (1993) 'Differences in illness intrusiveness across rheumatoid arthritis, end-stage renal disease, and multiple sclerosis', *Journal of Nervous and Mental Disease*, 181: 377–81.

Eisenberg, L. (1977) 'Disease and illness: Distinctions between professional and popular ideas of sickness', *Culture, Medicine and Psychiatry*, 1: 9–23.

Feinstein, A. (2004) 'The neuropsychiatry of multiple sclerosis', *Canadian Journal of Psychiatry*, 49: 157–63.

Finkelstein, V. (2001) *A Personal Journey into Disability Politics*. Leeds: The Disability Studies Archive UK, Centre for Disability Studies, University of Leeds.

Goffman, E. (1963) *Stigma: Notes on the Management of Spoiled Identity*. Englewood Cliffs, NJ: Prentice-Hall.

Goldberg, R. T. (1974) 'Adjustment of children with invisible and visible handicaps: Congenital heart disease and facial burns', *Journal of Counseling Psychology*, 21: 428–32.

Hennessey, A., Robertson, N.P., Swingler, R. and Compston, D.A.S. (1999) 'Urinary, faecal and sexual dysfunction in patients with multiple sclerosis', *Journal of Neurology*, 246: 1027–32.

Kos, D., Kerckhofs, E., Nagels, G., D'hooghe, M.B. and Ilsbroukx, S. (2008) 'Origin of fatigue in multiple sclerosis: Review of the literature', *Neurorehabilitation and Neural Repair*, 22: 91–100.

Mayo Clinic Staff (2009) *Multiple Sclerosis*. Mayo Foundation for Medical Education and Research (http://www.mayoclinic.com/health/multiple-sclerosis/DS00188).

Miserandino, C. (2010) *The Spoon Theory by Christine Miserandino: But You Don't Look Sick?* [Online]. Available at: http://www.butyoudontlooksick.com/articles/written-by-christine/the-spoon-theory-written-by-christine-miserandino/

Mitchell, A.J., Benito-León, J., González, J.-M.M. and Rivera-Navarro, J. (2005) 'Quality of life and its assessment in multiple sclerosis: Integrating physical and psychological components of wellbeing', *The Lancet Neurology*, 4: 556–66.

Multiple Sclerosis Encyclopaedia (2008) *Fatigue*. [Online]. Available at: http://www.mult-sclerosis.org/fatigue.html

Office for Disability Issues (2008) *Family Resources Survey (FRS) Disability Prevalence Estimates 2007/8*. London: Office for Disability Issues.

Office for National Statistics (2009) *Population: UK Population Aged 85 and Over Reaches 1.3 Million*. London: Office for National Statistics.

OPCS (2005) *National Statistics Online – Health and Wellbeing: More Years in Poor Health for Women*. London: Office for National Statistics.

Patten, S.B., Beck, C.A., Williams, J.V.A., Barbui, C. and Metz, L.M. (2003) 'Major depression in multiple sclerosis: A population-based perspective', *Neurology*, 61: 1524–7.

Patti, F. (2009) 'Cognitive impairment in multiple sclerosis', *Multiple Sclerosis*, 15: 2–8.

Reeve, D. (2002) 'Negotiating psycho-emotional dimensions of disability and their influence on identity constructions', *Disability & Society*, 17: 493–508.

Shakespeare, T. and Watson, N. (2002) 'The social model of disability: an outdated ideology?', *Exploring Theories and Expanding Methodologies: Research in Social Science and Disability*, 2: 9–28.

Siegert, R.J. and Abernethy, D.A. (2005) 'Depression in multiple sclerosis: a review', *Journal of Neurology, Neurosurgery & Psychiatry*, 76: 469–75.

Smith, C. and Hale, L. (2007) 'The unique nature of fatigue in multiple sclerosis: Prevalence, pathophysiology, contributing factors and subjective experience', *Physical Therapy Reviews*, 12: 43–51.

Sontag, S. (1978) *Illness as Metaphor*. London: Penguin.

Sprangers, M., De Regt, E., Andries, F., Van Agt, H., Bijl, R., De Boer, J., Foets, M., Hoeymans, N., Jacobs, A., Kempen, G., Miedema, H., Tijhuis, M. and De Haes, H. (2000) 'Which chronic conditions are associated with better or poorer quality of life?', *Journal of Clinical Epidemiology*, 53: 895–907.

Stone, S.D. (2005) 'Reactions to invisible disability: The experiences of young women survivors of hemorrhagic stroke', *Disability & Rehabilitation*, 27: 293–304.

Tam, S., Chan, M., Lam, H. and Lam, L. (2003) 'Comparing the self-concepts of Hong
     Kong Chinese adults with visible and not visible physical disability', *The Journal of
     Psychology: Interdisciplinary and Applied*, 137: 363–72.
UPIAS (1976) *Fundamental Principles of Disability*. Leeds: Leeds Disability Studies
     Archive [Online]. Available at: http://www.leeds.ac.uk/disability-studies/archiveuk/
     UPIAS/fundamental%20principles.pdf
Wendell, S. (2008) 'Notes from bed: Learning from chronic illness', in D. Driedger and
     M. Owen (eds), *Dissonant Disabilities: Women with Chronic Illnesses Explore Their Lives*.
     Toronto: Canadian Scholars' Press Inc / Women's Press.
White, C.P., White, M.B. and Russell, C.S. (2008) 'Invisible and visible symptoms of
     multiple sclerosis: Which are more predictive of health distress?', *Journal of
     Neuroscience Nursing*, 40: 85–95,102.
WHO (2002) *Towards a Common Language for Functioning, Disability and Health: ICF
     The International Classification of Functioning, Disability and Health*. Geneva: World
     Health Organization.

3

Experiencing Depression and Diabetes

Katharine Barnard and Cathy E. Lloyd

> ### Overview
>
> - Depression – how well is it understood?
> - The relationship between diabetes and depression
> - Overlap of the symptoms of depression and poorly controlled diabetes: the experiences of people with both these long-term conditions
> - Understanding the experience of depression and diabetes burnout
> - Health and social care in the context of depression
> - Challenges for practice

Depression is a term widely used but little understood. People often report feeling depressed when actually they're having a bad day or feeling low or fed up. Yet depression is a major, disabling illness affecting millions of people worldwide. The existing World Health Organization definition of depression is: 'a common mental disorder that presents with depressed mood, loss of interest or pleasure, feelings of guilt or low self-worth, disturbed sleep or appetite, low energy, and poor concentration'. It is a non-discriminatory disease in that it affects people of all genders, ages and backgrounds. Ranging from sub-clinical depressive symptomatology, at its worst depression can lead to suicide, contributing to an estimated 850,000 deaths worldwide every year (World Health Organization, 2010). Other important facts about depression include:

- it is very common, affecting 121 million people worldwide
- it is among the leading causes of disability worldwide
- it frequently occurs alongside other physical long-term conditions (e.g. heart disease or diabetes)
- it can be reliably diagnosed and treated in primary care, yet fewer than 25% of those affected have access to effective treatment. (World Health Organization, 2010)

Primary care based treatments for depression, although not universally available, are associated with improved quality of care, improved satisfaction with care, improved health functioning and outcomes and indirectly with improved economic productivity and household wealth. Such treatments, however, are firmly rooted in the medical model of care and rely heavily on the prescription of antidepressant medication, the effectiveness of which remains under debate (Fournier et al., 2010; Ionnidis, 2008).

People with diabetes have a greatly increased risk of mental health problems, especially depression (Lloyd et al., 2010; Schram et al., 2009); whilst at the same time having to grapple with the often perceived heavy burden of diabetes self-management. This combination of physical and mental health difficulties has led to serious challenges for the provision of appropriate care. This chapter will review the empirical evidence of increased rates of depression in this group as well as considering the more recent research on the impact of self-management on feelings of diabetes distress or 'burnout'. The difficulties of identifying whether an individual is feeling depressed or distressed and the implications for receiving health and social care will be debated.

Depression and depressive symptoms in people with diabetes

Current epidemiological evidence suggests that at least one third of people with diabetes also develop clinically relevant depressive disorders (Anderson et al., 2001; Barnard et al., 2006; Gendelman et al., 2009). The prevalence of depression in people with diabetes is significantly higher than that in the general population with people with diabetes being 2–3 times more likely to be considered to be depressed than their non-diabetic counterparts (Lloyd et al., 2010; Pouwer et al., 2010). Yet, depression may also increase the risk for diabetes (Nouwen et al., 2010) making the scenario very 'chicken and egg'. For example, one research study in the UK reported nearly a four-fold increased risk of diabetes in depressed men and a one-and-a-half times greater risk of diabetes in depressed women (Holt et al.,

2009). Furthermore, this latter study found that higher depression scores were associated with both diagnosed and undiagnosed diabetes, suggesting that the link between diabetes and depression does not solely result from the psychological distress experienced with the disease diagnosis. Clearly the relationship between diabetes and depression is complex and has yet to be fully understood.

Much of the recent research into diabetes and depression has focused on how having a physical disease (diabetes) can lead to poor mental health (depression). Pouwer and colleagues in the Netherlands have suggested that the unremitting practical and emotional burdens that often accompany diabetes self-management may play an important role and increase risk for depression (Pouwer et al., 2003). One potential focus for future research may be to address the personal burden of balancing diabetes (both medical and self-management components) with other competing demands on people's time, energy and workload in order to reduce this risk (Lloyd, 2010; Pouwer et al., 2003).

The other side of the coin is that depression can lead to poor self-care; in people with diabetes this could mean that their daily diabetes self-management might be affected, which may impact on blood sugar levels, potentially increasing the risk of developing diabetes-related complications (Katon et al., 2005; Kovacs and Obrosky, 1997; Lustman et al., 2000), and compromising quality of life (Schram et al., 2009). Low levels of depressive symptoms are also common, with an estimated prevalence ranging from 31% to 45% in people with diabetes (Gary et al., 2000; Hermanns et al., 2006). Thus, the association between depression and diabetes appears to be a vicious and spiralling potentially downwards cycle.

Both depression and diabetes are demanding long-term conditions that impact not only on the life of the individual, but also on the lives of other family members. Both conditions can interfere with normal functioning and can cause problems with work, social life and family relationships. For example, in one study, depression in people with diabetes was associated with increased physical health problems in their families (Sobieraj et al., 1998). Furthermore, in this study the burden of illness experienced by families of a depressed person was found to be far greater than that of families without a depressed member. Similarly, diabetes in at least one of the children can have a serious impact on the quality of life of other family members (Barnard et al., 2008). In this latter study, parents' self-reported quality of life was directly affected by the impact of their child's diabetes and treatment regime. This evidence of the psychological impact of diabetes on individuals and their families was acknowledged in the care recommendations laid out in the *National Service Framework for Diabetes* (DH,

2001: 22). Since then, the National Institute for Health and Clinical Excellence (NICE) has provided a framework in which to organize the provision of services for treating depression, supporting patients/carers and health care professionals in identifying and accessing the most effective interventions. However, there remain significant gaps in psychological services for people with diabetes which remain to be filled (Diabetes UK, 2005).

How are people with depression identified and diagnosed?

There are a number of tools available to measure the presence of symptoms of depression, as illustrated in the box below. Usually a screening tool might be used and then followed (if enough symptoms are present as measured by the screen) by a diagnostic interview. However given the lack of expertise in the field and poor provision of services, many more individuals are being identified as possibly depressed than there are opportunities for treatment and care which takes account of the psychosocial impact of depression. The majority of available screening tools measure the presence/absence of self-reported depressive symptoms (shown in the box below), and also the type and severity of those symptoms.

Symptoms of depression that may be measured in common self-report instruments used in both research and care

- Feeling sad/depressed mood
- Inability to sleep
- Early waking
- Lack of interest/enjoyment
- Tiredness/lack of energy
- Loss of appetite
- Feelings of guilt/worthlessness
- Recurrent thoughts about death/suicide

Validated and reliable measures for depression screening include the Center for Epidemiology Studies Depression (CES-D) scale, the Beck Depression Inventory (BDI) and the Patient Health Questionnaire (PHQ-9). All three of these instruments have been recommended by the National Institute of Health and Clinical Excellence (NICE) as appropriate for use in primary care in the UK (NICE, 2009). As most people with diabetes are cared for by their primary care physician it is in this setting that there are key opportunities for screening and providing care for people with mental health issues in their lives. A number of the screening tools have been evaluated by researchers to help practitioners have confidence that they identify people with depression (the sensitivity of the tool) rather than other conditions. Researchers have also considered whether or not tools over-estimate or over-diagnose cases of depression or whether they confuse symptoms of depression with somatic symptoms of physical disease (the specificity of the instrument). For clinical practice the positive and negative predictive values are also of considerable interest. A low positive predictive value is associated with a high rate of false positives (people identified as depressed who are actually not), and a low negative predictive value is associated with a high rate of false negatives (people considered not to be depressed who actually are). If the positive predictive value is low, the health care professional has to deal with numerous false positives, causing a lot of unnecessary additional diagnostic tests or referrals to mental health specialists.

Many screening tools contain both cognitive (thinking, reasoning) and somatic (physical) symptoms of depression and these may or may not overlap with some of the symptoms of diabetes, especially when diabetes control is poor or when the complications of diabetes (e.g. heart disease, diabetic retinopathy, kidney failure, peripheral neuropathy) start to develop. The overlapping symptoms include loss of/increase in appetite, difficulties sleeping, fatigue, loss of energy, and weight-loss. Cognitive symptoms may also be affected by diabetes; for example, fear of the future, hopelessness etc. It may be difficult therefore to disentangle reported symptoms which may relate to depression or to diabetes or even both. This is important because it may affect clinical decision-making, and treatment recommendations, as well as the individual service-user's experiences with health and social care.

The main limitation for most depression screening instruments is, unlike diagnostic interviews, the requirement for literacy unless the questionnaire is administered orally. It is also important to bear in mind when choosing which measure to use that there may be differences in the applicability of different screening instruments in particular sub-groups, for example in older people, in men or women, and in certain cultural or ethnic minority groups and for people for whom English is not their first language. In our recent research with South Asian people with diabetes, we asked focus group participants to describe how they felt and what the concept of depression meant to them. Some of their responses are shown in the box opposite.

What does depression mean to you?

'I think it is some sort of pain deep in your heart or pain in the head ... you can feel pain but it is difficult to explain to others'.

'It happens sometimes to me ... a feeling of tiredness and pain'.

'More or less a feeling of helplessness ... . It affects my daily activities'.

'Well I actually feel some kind of heaviness in my heart, when I am upset'.

Our research has highlighted some of the problems when trying to apply methods of assessing the symptoms of depression which have been developed for western English speaking people to individuals with different cultural backgrounds, languages or experiences. However there is beginning to be some progress in research and clinical practice which addresses these difficulties. Recently an international group of researchers and health care practitioners came together and formed the Dialogue on Diabetes and Depression (http://www.diabetesanddepression.org/), which aims to highlight the complexity of this issue and to develop research in this area.

The experience of distress: Is it depressive symptomatology or diabetes burnout?

Sub-clinical depression is a term used when individuals present with depressive symptoms but do not meet the criteria for a diagnosis of clinical depression. In some recent research conducted in the Netherlands, the authors (Pouwer and Hermanns, 2009) found that approximately one third of people with Type 1 diabetes and 37–43% of people with Type 2 diabetes reported symptoms of depression. These rates were far higher than the proportion of people who had been given an actual diagnosis of depression. However individuals with sub-clinical depression will very often not receive treatment but will cope with their symptoms alone. The impact of this in terms of effect on family, work and social life and overall quality of life remains unknown to a large extent and is an area where further research is clearly needed.

On the other hand, research has demonstrated that there are a substantial proportion of individuals who are not depressed and do not report depressive symptomatology, yet still feel unable to cope with their diabetes. It has been suggested that these people are experiencing diabetes-related distress or are 'burned out' by their diabetes. Diabetes burnout occurs when a person feels 'overwhelmed by diabetes and by the frustrating burden of diabetes self-care' (Polonsky et al., 1995). These emotions may be very different to feelings of depression; however they can still be very destructive and can have huge implications for care. Symptoms of burnout include:

- Feeling overwhelmed and defeated by diabetes
- Feeling angry about diabetes, frustrated by the self-care regimen and/or having other strong negative feelings about diabetes
- Feeling that diabetes is controlling their life
- Worrying about not taking care of diabetes well enough yet unable, unmotivated or unwilling to change
- Avoiding any/all diabetes related tasks that might give feedback about consequences of poor control
- Feeling alone and isolated with diabetes

Thus, whilst feelings of diabetes burnout centre on feelings about diabetes, depression is a physical and psychological disorder requiring specific medical attention. Consider the experiences of the two people in the case studies below; both describe symptoms of low mood and also diabetes-related distress or burnout. In both these scenarios it is the relationship between the person and their health care professional that is important, as the GP attempts to help the patient make sense of their distress and offer appropriate treatment.

Alan's story

Alan is 58 and has had Type 2 diabetes for 5 years. He works as an accounts manager for a local company selling cleaning products. He is a member of a local darts team and enjoys pottering round his garden during the weekend. Alan has strived to manage his diabetes over the years and until recently has not encountered any problems. However, two months ago he and his wife separated and he had to move out of the family home into a small flat a few miles away and only sees his two children at the weekends. Alan's blood sugar levels have started to fluctuate so at his appointment with his GP he voices his concerns. As he talks with his GP it becomes apparent to them both that Alan is feeling very sad and angry about his situation. He reveals that he has trouble sleeping, waking very early in the mornings, and has lost interest in his work and his hobbies. He reports feeling sad and tearful most of the time.

Alan's GP recognized his symptoms as signs of depression and, after further questioning, suggests he take a low-dose anti-depressant for a while.

Sarah's story

Sarah is 61 years old and has had Type 2 diabetes for 12 years. She used to take tablets for her diabetes but was advised a year ago by her GP to start insulin injections as her blood glucose levels were always too high. Sarah is married and has a grown-up daughter who is expecting her first child. She has recently retired from her job as a shop assistant as her eyesight is deteriorating and she was not able to drive to work.

Recently Sarah has been feeling quite anxious and has noticed that her blood sugar levels have started to fluctuate. At her next appointment with her GP she becomes upset; she says she feels like 'a failure', not being able to control her blood sugar levels and losing her eyesight. She worries constantly about her blood sugar levels and often tests her blood four or five times a day - not that she adjusted her insulin or anything, she just wants to reassure herself that they weren't too bad.

The doctor asked her what other things had been happening in her life recently, and she told him about giving up her job and that she didn't know what to do with herself all day and had resorted to 'comfort eating' in the evenings. After further questioning, Sarah's GP said he didn't think that she needed treatment for depression but that further support from the diabetes team might help her address her difficulties and help her feel less overwhelmed by her diabetes.

A key issue lies in the measurement of burnout or diabetes-related distress and the ability to disentangle these symptoms from those of depression. This has serious implications for care and any associated treatment or support. In the case studies above the GPs were able to assess the patient's distress by discussing symptoms and wider issues in their lives. Recently GPs have been able to use two simple screening questions to help them assess the possible presence of depressive symptoms (as opposed to diabetes-related distress or burnout). This may be followed by the use of the more precise screening tools discussed previously.

Screening questions for use in general practice

'During the past month have you often been bothered by feeling down, depressed or hopeless?'

'During the past month have you often been bothered by little interest or pleasure in doing things?'

(Arroll et al., 2003; Whooley et al., 2008).

Whilst these two screening questions may be easily administered and quite easily answered by many people attending their GP, this may not be the case for all. In our research with South Asian people we noted some confusion and misunderstanding about these two questions as well as some quite critical comments on their use in people whose first or main language is not English:

> 'When it is in English we do not understand many terms. I think it is important to ask this type of question. But the problem is … it needs to be clear and understandable to us … only then can we answer properly.'

> 'The GPs ask many things … sometimes they just ask this type of question without explaining anything. It looks like they have loads of paper work and their target is to finish everything during consultation. Sometimes they do not have enough time to explain I think.'

When one participant had to use an interpreter when going to his GP he reported even more problems:

> 'I did not find even the interpreter explaining things to me properly. They just translate … something that the GP wanted to know and then will translate that back to the GP in a language I don't understand at all. I actually don't know what is going on between them … or even if they are translating my right feelings to the GP.'

Notwithstanding these problems, as discussed earlier there are widely accepted methods for measuring depression and depressive symptomatology, however it is less easy to identify the symptoms of diabetes-related burnout. There are a number of resources available to help both practitioners and individuals with diabetes identify whether they are 'burned out' (Polonsky et al., 1995, 2005), however there are no official recommendations or clinical guidelines which require health care practitioners to use them to help inform the care they provide for people with diabetes. Some research has indicated that there may be particular people who are at greater risk of experiencing diabetes-distress, for example women, those with diabetes complications and individuals who report negative life-events (Fisher et al., 2009). There may be serious implications for care too – research suggests those with diabetes-distress also have poor diabetic control (Polonsky et al., 1995). Clearly, it is important to try to identify those people experiencing diabetes-distress and address the health and social care needs of those individuals.

Health and social care in the context of depression

Diabetes has a significant impact on health and social care services (Sampson et al., 2006). People with diabetes are twice as likely to be admitted to hospital as those without diabetes and people with diabetes experience prolonged stays in hospital. This results in about 80,000 additional bed days per year in the UK (Sampson et al., 2006). The presence of diabetic complications increases NHS costs more than five-fold and increases five-fold the chance of a person needing hospital admission. One in 20 people with diabetes also incurs social services costs. In one report more than three-quarters of these costs were associated with residential and nursing care, while home help services accounted for a further one-fifth (Sampson et al., 2006). The presence of complications increases social services costs four-fold (Kings Fund, 2000).

The personal cost of diabetes may be lost within these financial figures, however research has clearly demonstrated that diabetes has a direct impact on individual social functioning and quality of life (Barnard et al., 2007). The impact on family members, relationships and the ability to interact with friends and colleagues should not be underestimated (Hislop et al., 2007; Lloyd et al., 1993). This can include relatives not wanting to leave the house for fear of 'not being there', for example in some research looking at the impact of diabetes, one woman reported not wanting to leave her husband alone in the house in case 'he has a hypo whilst I'm out and I'm not there to help him' (Barnard et al., 2007) Another participant reported that following a change in insulin therapy her 'mum doesn't go into meltdown at family weddings' any more because she was worried about content and timing of food. Perhaps the real cost of diabetes is not measured in monetary terms, but rather in terms of the impact that it has on people's ability to go about their daily lives and enjoy life's pleasures. People with diabetes have a worse quality of life than people without chronic illness (Rubin and Peyrot, 1999) but a better quality of life than people with most other serious long-term conditions. The picture is rather complex however, and it is not clear whether quality of life is most affected in those with diabetes of long duration or whether those with a particular type of diabetes or treatment regimen have a poorer life quality. For example, continuous subcutaneous insulin therapy (CSII) is widely reported to improve life quality for individuals with Type 1 diabetes and their family members (Barnard et al., 2007, 2008). Having better blood glucose control is associated with better quality of life (Rubin and Peyrot, 1999), yet a person's ability to engage in appropriate self-care behaviours is significantly impaired when they suffer from depression as well as diabetes (Lloyd et al., 2010). Complications of diabetes are the most important disease-specific determinant of quality of life.

Although more studies are needed, research has shown that diabetes education to support self-management has a positive impact on diabetes and can help improve quality of life. The *National Service Framework for*

Diabetes recommended a partnership approach to diabetes care (Department of Health, 2001), which implies that health care professionals and the person with diabetes should work together towards commonly agreed goals in order to optimize care and improve outcomes. The principle of empowerment in diabetes care is based upon people taking more control of their care, both for themselves as individuals, and also for others being involved in determining local services and priorities (Anderson and Funnell, 2000). An empowerment approach to care takes into account social, psychological and environmental factors as well as medical ones. So, for example, when a health care worker provides advice on diet, they must consider that food does more than simply satisfy hunger, rather foods have cultural, interpersonal and emotional meanings that must be understood to negotiate a realistic nutrition plan for diabetes self-management (Anderson and Rubin, 2002). It is pointless trying to prescribe an eating plan that cannot realistically be achieved due to social, cultural or environmental factors.

Challenging existing practice

Depression is costly to the NHS in financial terms, with prescriptions per head for all antidepressants increasing 2.8-fold between 1991 and 2002, and the total cost (adjusted for inflation) increasing by £310m (Hollinghurst et al., 2005). The prescribing of antidepressant drugs has increased significantly in recent years; whilst at the same time there have been growing concerns about the medicalization of human distress and the safety of antidepressant medication (Gunnell and Ashby, 2004). Prescribed medication for depression has been the mainstay of treatment for depression in general practice despite the availability of alternative non-pharmacological psychological therapies such as cognitive behavioural therapy. Increases in the pharmacological treatment of depression have not been matched by the development of psychological services of proved effectiveness (Hollinghurst et al., 2005).

Despite the clinical and cost effectiveness of psychological therapies such as cognitive behavioural therapy (CBT) (Ismail et al., 2010), existing practice in the NHS remains predominantly pharmacological. There are currently no formal clinical pathways for delivering expert psychological care specifically for people with diabetes (Nicholson et al., 2009). However, both the National Service Framework (NSF) and the National Institute for Health and Clinical Excellence (NICE) have made explicit recommendations and set standards to provide counselling (NSF standard 3) and management of depression (NSF standard 12). Broader guidance for the treatment of depression in people with a range of long-term conditions has now been published by NICE (2009), but at the time of writing remains in the consultation process.

In a study conducted in diabetes centres throughout the UK, Nicholson and his colleagues (2009) reported that less than a third of responding centres (n = 84) had access to specialist psychological services. Availability of such services was variable across the four UK nations. Over two thirds of centres had not implemented the majority of national guidelines, with under 3% meeting all guidelines. Yet despite such a sparse availability of psychological support, provision of psychological input into teams was associated with 'the perception of better skills in managing more complex psychological issues, increased likelihood of having psychological care pathways and improved training in psychological issues for team members' (Nicholson et al., 2009: 447).

In spite of more research in the field, the availability of guidance for care and increased support for psychological care for people with long-term conditions, health care workers continue to be constrained by an emphasis on biomedical outcomes. However there are moves to also consider the emotional and psychosocial impact of diabetes. The growing numbers of multidisciplinary teams in primary care, providing holistic support to patients and greater use of talking therapies could reduce the diabetes burden. Greater links between research and practice, where health care professionals work more closely with researchers would enable the findings of research to be utilized in a more immediate way.

Summary

Depression is common in people with diabetes, and represents a costly and burdensome condition, both in financial and psychosocial terms. The mechanisms of the relationship between symptoms of depression and diabetes require further exploration, with the question of how best to support people with both these long-term conditions remaining an important area of clinical care and research. It is clear that a move away from the orthodox medical model of care is insufficient to provide adequate and appropriate support and complimentary psychological therapies such as talking therapies have a greater role to play in this regard. Antidepressant prescribing alone is not enough to address the complex and often competing demands of diabetes and depression. This would require a shift in medical practice from didactic one-to-one GP consultations to a greater emphasis on multidisciplinary team working and greater use of talking therapies alongside traditional pharmacological ones.

Further reading

Katon, W., Maj, M. and Sartorius, N. (eds) (2010) *Depression and Diabetes.* Oxford: John Wiley.

Khunti, K., Kumar, S. and Brodie, J. (eds) (2009) *Diabetes UK and South Asian Health Foundation Recommendations on Diabetes Research Priorities for British South Asians.* London: Diabetes UK.

Lloyd, C.E. (2010) 'Diabetes and mental health; the problem of co-morbidity', *Diabetic Medicine,* 27: 853–4.

NICE (2009) *Depression in Adults with a Chronic Physical Health Problem* [Online]. Available at: http://www.nice.org.uk/nicemedia/live/12327/45865/45865.pdf (accessed 15 October 2010).

References

Anderson, R.M. and Funnell, M.M. (2000) *The Art of Empowerment.* Alexandria: American Diabetes Association.

Anderson, B.J., and Rubin, R. (eds.). (2002) *Practical Psychology for Diabetes Clinicians* (2nd edn). Alexandria: American Diabetes Association.

Anderson R.J., Freedland, K.E., Klaus, R.E. and Lustman, P.J. (2001) 'The prevalence of comorbid depression in adults with diabetes: A meta-analysis', *Diabetes Care,* 24(6): 1069–78.

Arroll, B., Khin, N. and Kerse, N. (2003) 'Screening for depression in primary care with two verbally asked questions: cross sectional study', *British Medical Journal,* 327: 1144–6.

Barnard, K.D., Skinner, T.C. and Peveler, R. (2006) 'The prevalence of comorbid depression in adults with Type 1 diabetes', *Diabetic Medicine,* 23(4): 445–8.

Barnard, K.D., Lloyd, C.E. and Skinner, T.C. (2007) 'Systematic literature review into quality of life issues surrounding insulin pump use in Type 1 diabetes', *Diabetic Medicine,* 24(6): 607–17.

Barnard, K.D., Speight, J. and Skinner, T.C. (2008) 'Quality of life and impact of continuous subcutaneous insulin infusion for children and their parents', *Practical Diabetes International,* 25(7): 278–84.

Department of Health (DH) (2001) *National Service Framework for Diabetes.* London: Department of Health.

Diabetes UK (2005) *State of the Nations 2005: Progress made in Delivering the National Diabetes Frameworks* [Online]. Available at: http://www.diabetes.nhs.uk/downloads/StateOfNations.pdf (accessed 15 October 2010).

Fisher, L., Mullan, J.T., Skaff, M.M., Glasgow, R.E., Arean, P. and Hessler, D. (2009) 'Predicting diabetes distress in patients with Type 2 diabetes: A longitudinal study', *Diabetic Medicine,* 26: 622–7.

Fournier, J., DeRubeis, R.J., Hollon, S.D., Dimidjian, S., Amsterdam, J.D., Shelton, R.C. and Fawcett, J. (2010) 'Antidepressant drug effects and depression severity', *JAMA,* 303: 47–53.

Gary, T.L., Crum, R.M., Cooper-Patrick, L., Ford, D. and Brancati, F.L. (2000) 'Depressive symptoms and metabolic control in African-Americans with Type 2 diabetes', *Diabetes Care,* 23(1): 23–9.

Gendelman, N., Snell-Bergeon, J.K., McFann, K., Kinney, G., Wadwa, R.P., Bishop, F., Rewers, M. and Maahs, D.M. (2009) 'Prevalence and correlates of depression in individuals with and without Type 1 diabetes', *Diabetes Care*, 32(4): 575–9.

Gunnell, D. and Ashby, D. (2004) 'Antidepressants and suicide: What is the balance of benefit and risk?', *British Medical Journal*, 329: 34–8.

Hermanns, N., Kulzer, B., Krichbaum, M., Kubiak, T. and Haak, T. (2006) How to screen for depression and emotional problems in patients with diabetes: Comparison of screening characteristics of depression questionnaires, measurement of diabetes-specific emotional problems and standard clinical assessment', *Diabetologia*, 49(3): 469–77.

Hislop, A.L., Fegan, P.G., Schaeppi, M.J., Duck, M. and Yeap, B.B. (2007) 'Prevalence and associations of psychological distress in young adults with Type 1 diabetes', *Diabetic Medicine*, 25(1): 91–6.

Hollinghurst, S., Kesseler, D., Peters, T.J. and Gunnell, D. (2005) 'Opportunity cost of antidepressant prescribing in England: Analysis of routine data', *British Medical Journal*, 330.[Online] Available at BMJ2005;330:999doi:10.1136/bmj.38377.715799. F7 (accessed 15 October 2010).

Holt, R.I.G., Phillips, W., Jameson, K.A., Cooper, C., Dennison, E.M. and Peveler, R.C. (2009) 'Education and psychological aspects: The relationship between depression and diabetes mellitus: findings from the Hertfordshire Cohort Study', *Diabetic Medicine*, 26: 641–8.

Ionnidis, J. (2008) 'Effectiveness of antidepressants: An evidence myth constructed from a thousand randomised trials?', *Philosophy, Ethics, and Humanities in Medicine*, 3: 14.

Ismail, K., Thomas, S., Chalder, T., Schmidt, U., Bartlett, J., Patel, A., Dickens, C., Creed, F. and Treasure, J. (2010) 'A randomised controlled trial of cognitive behaviour therapy and motivational interviewing for people with Type 1 diabetes mellitus with persistent sub-optimal glycaemic control: A Diabetes and Psychological Therapies (ADaPT) study', *Health Technology Assessment (Winchester, England)*, 14(22): 1–101, iii–iv.

Katon, W. J., Rutter, C., Simon, G., Lin, E., Ludman, E., Ciechanowski, P., Kinder, L., Young, B. and von Korff, M. (2005) 'The association of comorbid depression with mortality in patients with Type 2 diabetes', *Diabetes Care*, 28(11): 2668–72.

Kings Fund (2000) 'Tardis: Type 2 diabetes: accounting for major resource demand in society in the UK', *Diabetic Medicine*, 23 (9): 1008–15.

Kovacs, M. and Obrosky, D.S. (1997) 'Major depressive disorder in youths with IDDM. A controlled prospective study of course and outcome', *Diabetes Care*, 20(1): 45–51.

Lloyd, C.E. (2010) 'Diabetes and mental health: The problem of co-morbidity', *Diabetic Medicine Editorial*, 27: 853–4.

Lloyd C.E., Robinson, N., Elston, M.A., Andrews, B., Fuller, J.H. (1993) 'Are the social relationships of young insulin-dependent diabetic patients affected by illness?', *Diabetic Medicine*, 10: 481–5.

Lloyd, C.E., Hermanns, N., Nouwen, A., Pouwer, F., Underwood, L. and Winkley, K. (2010) 'The epidemiology of depression and diabetes', in W. Katon, M. Maj and N. Sartorius (eds), *Depression and Diabetes*. Oxford: Wiley-Blackwell.

Lustman, P.J., Anderson, R.J., Freedland, K.E., de Groot, M., Carney, R.M. and Clouse, R.E. (2000) 'Depression and poor glycemic control: A meta-analytic review of the literature', *Diabetes Care*, 23(7): 934–42.

NICE (2009) *Depression in Adults with a Chronic Physical Health Problem* [Online]. Available at: http://www.nice.org.uk/nicemedia/live/12327/45865/45865.pdf (accessed 15 October 2010).

Nicholson, T.R.J., Taylor, J.P., Gosden, C., Trigwell, P. and Ismail, K. (2009) 'National guidelines for psychological care in diabetes: how mindful have we been?', *Diabetic Medicine*, 26: 447–50 .

Nouwen, A., Winkley, K., Twisk, J., Lloyd, C.E., Peyrot, M., Ismail, K. and Pouwer, F. for the European Depression in Diabetes (EDID) Research Consortium (2010) 'Type 2 Diabetes Mellitus as a risk factor for the onset of depression: a systematic review and meta-analysis', *Diabetologia*, 53(12): 2480–6.

Polonsky, W., Anderson, B., Lohrer, .P, Welch, G., Jacobson, A. and Aponte, J. (1995) 'Assessment of diabetes related distress', *Diabetes Care*, 18: 754–60.

Polonsky, W. H., Fisher, L. et al. (2005) 'Assessing psychosocial distress in diabetes: development of the diabetes distress scale', *Diabetes Care*, 28(3): 626–31.

Pouwer, F. and Hermanns, N. (2009) 'Insulin therapy and quality of life. A review', *Diabetes Metabolism Research*, 25 Suppl 1: S4–S10.

Pouwer, F., Beekman, T.F., Nijpels, G., Dekker, J.M., Snoek, P.J., Kostense, R.J., Heine, D.J. and Deeg, D.J.H. (2003) 'Rates and risks for comorbid depression in patients with Type 2 diabetes mellitus: results from a community-based study', *Diabetologia*, 46; 892–8.

Pouwer, F., Geelhoed-Duijveestihn, H.L.M., Tack, C.J., Bazelmans, E., Beekman, A-J., Heine, R.J. and Snoek, F.J. (2010) 'Prevalence of comorbid depression is high in out-patients with Type 1 or Type 2 diabetes mellitus. Results from the three out-patient clinics in the Netherlands', *Diabetic Medicine*, 27: 217–24.

Rubin, R. and Peyrot, M. (1999) 'Quality of life and diabetes', *Diabetes/Metabolism Research and Reviews*, 15: 205–18.

Sampson, M.J., Crowle, T., Dhatariya, K., Dozio, N., Greenwood, R.H., Heyburn, P.J., Jones, C., Temple, R.C. and Walden, E. (2006) 'Trends in bed occupancy for inpatients with diabetes before and after the introduction of a diabetes inpatient specialist nurse service', *Diabetic Medicine*, 23(9): 1008–15.

Schram, M.T., Baan, C.A. and Pouwer, F. (2009) 'Depression and quality of life in patients with diabetes: A systematic review from the European depression in diabetes (EDID) research consortium', *Current Diabetes Review*, 5(2): 112–19.

Sobieraj, M., Williams, J. and Ryan, P. (1998) 'The impact of depression on the physical health of family members', *British Journal of General Practice*, 48(435): 1653–5.

Whooley, M.A., de Jonge, P., Vittinghoff, E., Otte, C., Moos, R., Carney, R.M., Ali, S., Dowray, S., Na, B., Feldman, M.D., Schiller, N.B. and Browner, W.S. (2008) 'Depressive symptoms, health behaviors, and risk of cardiovascular events in patients with coronary heart disease', *Journal of the American Medical Association*, 300(20): 2379–88.

World Health Organization (2010) [Online] Available at: http://www.who.int/en/ (accessed 2 October 2010).

4

Experiencing and Managing Medically Unexplained Conditions: The Case of Chronic Pelvic Pain in Women

Elaine Denny

Overview

- Chronic pelvic pain (CPP) is a debilitating gynaecological condition in women, which impacts on quality of life
- For many women with CPP a clinical diagnosis is never reached, and they are left with unsatisfactory explanations for their pain
- Having pain defined as 'unexplained' has an impact on social relationships and interactions with health professionals
- Within the medical profession CPP is viewed as a difficult condition which could have many different causes, and is often accompanied by assumptions of psychological disturbance or previous sexual abuse

Definition and epidemiology

Chronic pelvic pain is a debilitating condition in women, which impacts on quality of life and costs the NHS an estimated £158 million per annum

(Latthe et al., 2006). It is usually considered to be a gynaecological condition, and it is only in recent years that a label of CPP has been applied to chronic prostatitis in men. CPP is usually defined as noncyclical pelvic or lower abdominal pain of more than 3 or 6 months duration, that may be intermittent or continuous. Some definitions also include the lack of pathology, but there is no standardized definition and the notion of a 'woman's problem' has influenced the research that is conducted on the issue. Williams et al. (2004: 686) argue that 'the use of a poor operational chronic pelvic pain research definition reduces the ability to investigate causation and improve treatment of this condition'. Despite this lack of definition gynaecologists Khalid Khan and Pallavi Latthe (2009) state that CPP is characterized by an ill-defined onset, unpredictable duration, persistence, commonly accompanied by depression, and not usually helped by rest. Some commentators seek to differentiate CPP from cyclic pain and dysmenorrhoea, but as Victoria Grace, a sociologist, and psychologist Sara MacBride-Stewart (2007) found in their qualitative study for many women it is not possible to clearly differentiate pain with and without menstruation.

Each year approximately 38 in 1,000 women attend primary care services for CPP, and in community surveys 15–24% of women aged between 18 and 50 years report experiencing it within the previous three months (McGowan et al., 2010). A systematic review on the international incidence of CPP suggests a prevalence rate for non-cyclic CPP in the UK of 24%, and internationally a range of 4–43.4% (Latthe et al., 2006). The authors suggest that the international differences may be due to study characteristics and quality, definitions used and age groups included rather than intrinsic differences in incidence. Another factor that will be discussed within the chapter is that various ethnic groups may interpret the experience of CPP differently and this may affect the way it is managed by women in various parts of the world.

Although it has a rate of GP consultation similar to asthma or back pain CPP remains a poorly understood condition (McGowan et al., 2010). Investigations such as ultrasound scans or laparoscopy may elicit a diagnosis of endometriosis or adhesions, and endocervical swabs may identify pelvic infection, but for many women their pain remains unexplained within a biomedical framework. It is the impact of this lack of medical diagnosis and of the label 'unexplained chronic pelvic pain' on the experience of CPP that I will explore in this chapter, and offer some suggestions for improving the care of women with CPP within the health system.

The importance of diagnosis

In order to understand why unexplained CPP is so problematic it is useful to explore the importance of a diagnosis in modern health care. Science historian Charles Rosenburg reminds us that diagnosis has always played a pivotal role in medical practice, but that over the past two centuries as medicine (in line with society more generally) has become more technical, specialized and bureaucratic, its role has become more central. 'Diagnosis labels, defines, and predicts and, in doing so, helps constitute and legitimate the reality that it discerns' (Rosenburg, 2002: 240). By receiving a diagnosis a person is accepted as genuinely ill, because an impartial expert has given them legitimacy and a label that encompasses an explanation for their symptoms. The recent advent and proliferation of diagnostic procedures has increased the apparent certainty with which a diagnosis can be offered, matching expressed symptoms with some form of visible pathology within the body, or providing a quantitative measure that can be compared to an accepted norm. Failure to reach a diagnosis is no longer an acceptable option for patients, and rather than accept the infallibility of the technology doctors may question the credibility of the patient. Medical training instils in doctors an imperative to reach a diagnosis (Denny, 2009), to replace the uncertainty of a collection of symptoms by the structure of a disease label. A diagnosis sets in train a trajectory for interventions, treatment, and hopefully a cure for the disease, or at least a predictable prognosis for the future. A lack of diagnosis may be followed by a more *ad hoc* response to individual symptoms at best, or at worst suspicions of malingering, exaggeration or hypochondria by both health professionals and the family and friends of the sufferer.

However receiving a diagnosis is not necessarily unproblematic. Grace and MacBride-Stewart (2007) found that some women questioned the diagnosis they had been given, such as cysts and haemorrhoids, either because they were unsure that cysts or haemorrhoids were actually present, or because they did not accept them as an explanation for the pain.

Recently a label of medically unexplained symptoms (MUS) has been applied to some patients, which sociologist Sarah Nettleton states includes 'those patients who have symptoms that have no identified organic basis' (2006: 1168). She further notes that this was initially a description rather than a label, but there is now an attempt to differentiate between those people with MUS who have mental health problems and are classified as 'somatizers' and those who do not (Nettleton, 2006). However many references are made to psychosocial factors among the latter group, and Sharpe defines MUS as 'symptoms that are disproportionate to identifiable physical disease' (Sharpe, 2001: 501). This implies that an objective judgement can be made about correct or appropriate levels of pain for specific diseases or level of pathology. In reality such judgements are highly subjective (Denny, 2009). Bendelow (2009) argues that the label MUS is less stigmatizing than 'psychosomatic illness', but as it describes illness that cannot be explained in terms of pathology it is low in importance in the medical hierarchy of disease. Many people in Nettleton's study of neurological symptoms did not necessarily want a diagnosis, accepting that medicine is not always clear cut, but they did want their symptoms acknowledged as genuine. People also want an explanation or, as Grace and MacBride-Stewart (2007) argue, an answer to 'how come' they have this pain.

Pain and gender

More women than men report experiencing chronic pain, and a greater number of chronic pain conditions have a higher female prevalence (Grace and Zondervan, 2006). More women than men seek treatment for chronic pain (Bendelow and Williams, 2000). However these figures may in part be the result of the gendered classification mentioned above. Much research on gender and pain has found that women are assumed to have a higher pain threshold and to be able to cope with pain better than men, but Bendelow and Williams (2000) looked beyond these beliefs to consider why they were held. They found that within their sample of men and women the reproductive role was believed to equip women with a natural capacity to endure pain both physically and emotionally. Pain was also viewed as being part of a woman's healthy life, whereas men were seen as experiencing pain only during illness or injury. Men were also seen as more stoical as a result of socialization into a role where they are supposed to be strong and not display emotion. The consequence of these assumptions is a further assumption that women can put up with more pain and that their pain does not need to be taken so seriously. Bendelow and Williams (2000) argue that for men and women gendered notions of pain are a double edged sword, and the experience of CPP, in particular in women's encounters with health professionals, is certainly influenced by gender.

Whether CPP is associated with menstruation or not, an association is frequently made with hormonal changes and the idea that it is a normal part of being a woman. So some women in Grace and MacBride-Stewart's study (2007: 55) spoke of pain in relation to being 'out-of-kilter' and having overactive hormones. However, the use of the word 'normal' here was not the same as the normal/pathological dualism of biomedical discourse, rather normal pain was viewed by women as something that all women get. Moreover, health psychologist Linda McGowan and colleagues (2010) argue that the reliance on laparoscopy to assign women into pathological or non-pathological categories reduces complex pain phenomena to a simplistic dualist model. This is compounded by a stereotype of a CPP patient as a sexually abused or depressed woman, all of which adds up to a poor experience within health services. This may then limit the management options considered. However, women themselves are influenced by the dominant biomedical model and have high expectations that a laparoscopy will provide a cause for their pain, and feel confused and anxious when the results are not consistent with their sense of something being wrong. Women in the studies by both Savidge et al. (1998) and McGowan et al. (2010) talk of feeling 'stuck' when laparoscopy fails to produce an explanation for their pain, unable (or not entitled) to return to health services even though their pain persists.

The experience of CPP

The management of women with CPP in primary care has been shown to be frustrating for both women and health professionals. Lack of a satisfactory explanation results in many women embarking on the so-called medical merry go round. Negative investigation results are followed by referral to different specialists and another set of investigations. Women have also been accused of 'doctor shopping' but this pejorative term belies the trauma that women experience when they are disbelieved or 'fobbed off', a term that is used frequently within women's stories. Women in one study felt obliged to justify their pain as they felt they were not believed by doctors, particularly if they were not actually experiencing pain during the consultation (Savidge et al., 1998). The end of the line is often referral to a pain clinic, which may be perceived by women in a negative light, as there being nothing left in terms of a cure, rather than being a positive opportunity for managing their pain.

McGowan et al. (2010) reported that the GPs in their study showed sensitivity to women, and stressed the importance of taking women seriously and believing what they say. However, professed behaviour is frequently reported in terms that are consistent with ideal or acceptable behaviour, and there was also an underlying moral discourse that blamed a woman's lifestyle for her symptoms. One GP described women with CPP as 'miserable and depressed with poor sex lives', and they were generally viewed as difficult to manage (McGowan et al., 2010: 312). McGowan et al. (1999) state that this type of description fails to delineate a causal mechanism or to consider that constant pain, often unexplained, may lead to depression and sexual difficulties rather than being the cause.

Women with CPP are often included in the group of patients labelled 'heartsink'. This term was first used in the late 1980s by Nottingham GP Tom O'Dowd to describe those patients who 'evoke an overwhelming mixture of exasperation, defeat and sometimes plain dislike that causes the heart to sink when they consult' (O'Dowd, 1988: 528). It is the doctor or other health professional who decides that a patient meets these criteria; patients are rarely given the opportunity to challenge the assumptions that underpin the label. Heartsink patients tend to be thought of as those with psychosomatic illness, lower social class, female, having thick clinical records, and making frequent use of the health services. Butler and Evans (1999) add persistent visits to the doctor, unresolved clinical symptoms and difficulties in defining a clinical problem. Women with undiagnosed CPP will fulfil some of these conditions, and by viewing them as heartsink patients the problem is transferred from being a failure of individual doctors or the biomedical system to treat them satisfactorily, to being a weakness or moral failing within the patient.

Qualitative research on the experience of CPP has been carried out by, amongst others, Savidge et al. (1998) and Grace and MacBride-Stewart (2007). A quantitative study has been conducted by Grace and Zondervan (2006). The findings from qualitative studies are consistent and describe women's relentless struggles with pain, often over many years. Findings from a population-based study support the data from qualitative research (Grace and Zondervan, 2006). CPP often has no pattern and is unpredictable, but whatever the cycle of pain/no pain it affects all aspects of a woman's life. It is also very isolating, as people do not understand it and the lack of diagnosis leads family and friends, and often the woman herself, to question whether the pain is real. Savidge et al. (1998) report women experiencing depression brought on by the effects of the pain and by not being believed. In their population-based study comparing the health of women with CPP, dysmenorrhoea only, dyspareunia (pain on intercourse) with no pelvic pain, or no pain, Grace and Zondervan (2006) found that women with CPP or dyspareunia had worse general health, more sleep disturbance and a greater incidence of other long standing illnesses than the other groups.

This body of work also reveals the many coping strategies that women employ in order to keep going within their multiple roles as workers, mothers and so on, for example by planning ahead in terms of pain relief or the timing of outings. However, CPP affects a woman's life physically, socially and emotionally and women in the study by Savidge et al. (1998) often compared their lives before experiencing CPP to their current life. For example, one woman who had been very active and played many sports had had to curtail these activities due to pain or to the fear of pain starting at a time or place where it could not be dealt with. Other women described CPP as 'emotionally draining', 'it turns your life upside down', 'it makes you miserable' (Savidge et al., 1998: 110).

In a study that recruited women with CPP via a newspaper advertisement McGowan et al. (2007) report that women who have repeated unsatisfactory encounters with health professionals may disengage with formal health services. Participants wrote their stories following a loose topic guide provided by the researchers and the narratives produced suggested that certain factors could stop the flow of the diagnostic cycle and lead women to disengage with mainstream services. Things said during consultations that lead women to feel that their story (their reality) was not believed provided a powerful trigger to disengagement, particularly after repeated attempts to have their story heard were rejected. Women felt powerless, and reluctant to set themselves up for further rejection. The way that women were told about negative test results could also lead them to disengage. This is consistent with Savidge et al. (1998) who found that 18 months after a negative laparoscopy the majority of their sample was still experiencing pain, but not receiving medical care. Women in both studies were seeking if not a diagnosis then recognition that their pain was real, and being told that nothing was found in such a way that implied that the pain was exaggerated left many women feeling frustrated and also anxious that something serious could have been missed. McGowan et al. (2007) differentiate this type of disengagement from a more deliberate exit strategy that can give people a sense of control. Rather this was a passive process undertaken by women who had been on the 'medical merry go round', 'felt stuck' and could not face another encounter that invalidated their pain. Despite these negative encounters with health professionals much research (e.g. Denny, 2009; Savidge et al., 1998) finds that women's criticisms are directed at individual health professionals, usually doctors, and not seen as a generalized failure of biomedicine, even though as Bendelow (2009: 58) argues biomedicine has traditionally been unable to deal adequately with those patients that she describes as being in 'diagnostic limbo'.

Once disengaged, women may try complementary therapies such as acupuncture or homeopathy or self-help measures, for example a TENS machine or application of heat. They may just live with the pain until some trigger encourages them to attempt further investigations and treatments. So the number of women known to health services may comprise a clinical iceberg that is the visible minority of a group of women who are much greater in number. The women who suffer in silence may be hidden from research into CPP which tends to recruit participants from clinics or self-help groups, and their stories go unheard.

In a similar vein, little work has been carried out with women with pelvic pain from minority ethnic groups, or on the influence of cultural factors in seeking professional help for CPP. One study that looked at the experiences of endometriosis (the commonest known cause of pelvic pain) and its treatment with five minority ethnic communities provides insight into the barriers that some women can face when suffering from gynaecological conditions (Denny et al., 2010). Women whose families originated in the Indian subcontinent spoke of the expectation that marriage would quickly lead to pregnancy, as producing children was seen as the main purpose of marriage. Any suspicion that a woman may have problems in conceiving, however unfounded, may affect her prospects of marriage. A gynaecological problem can raise concern in the family of a prospective husband, and women would rather endure pain than affect their chances of marriage. For Pakistani and, to a lesser extent, Indian women in the study, virginity at marriage was very important. Interventions that are routine in gynaecology such as internal examinations and the use of oral contraception as front line treatment, can raise suspicions of sexual activity and render a woman unmarriageable within her community, which is highly stigmatizing for her and her family. These two issues make women, particularly unmarried women, reluctant to seek medical treatment for their pain, and may help to explain the relatively low numbers of South Asian women seen in endometriosis clinics. Similar barriers may exist for other groups of women who may then contribute to the clinical iceberg of CPP.

Sexual abuse

A link between previous sexual abuse and CPP in adulthood has been postulated by a number of authors, for example Lampe et al. (2000) and Randolph and Reddy (2006). However there are frequently methodological problems with such research. As stated above there is no standard definition of CPP and a study of definitions used in peer reviewed, published primary research on CPP found that 95% of definitions did not consider co-morbidity, which may seriously impact on any relationship between CPP and a history of abuse (Williams et al., 2004). Similarly there is no agreed definition of sexual abuse, and while any unwanted sexual attention may be defined as sexual abuse, in reality what constitutes this will differ between women. When comparing women with CPP with women with other types of chronic pain, the appropriateness of the control group is often questionable and the recruitment of controls vague. Lampe et al. (2000) used healthy women attending primary care for routine checks as controls, and it is possible that this group of women may have been less willing to speak freely about sexual abuse. Frequent gynaecological examinations and consultations, which will be more common among women with CPP than healthy controls, may bring to the fore incidents from childhood that others keep repressed.

History of sexual abuse is often ascertained using self-report questionnaires, which do not tease out the relationship between CPP, current sexual difficulties and previous sexual abuse. Response rate to these questionnaires may be low, for example only 43 out of 63 women in the study by Poleshuck et al. (2005) responded to questions about abuse. Of these 15 (23.8% of the total sample) reported at least one incidence of sexual abuse. Moreover, questionnaires may ask about experiences that range from 'unwanted touching' to 'rape' but researchers do not always differentiate in reporting the results, and may reduce various types of experience to an abused/not abused dichotomy (Randolph and Reddy, 2006). Recruitment of women tends to be from pain clinics or tertiary centres and these women may have more complex experience and pathology, including a greater history of previous sexual abuse. Samples are therefore not representative of the many women who are managed within primary care or who self-manage.

Pitts et al. (2000) take a historical view of CPP and offer some explanation as to why the association with sexual abuse has become so ubiquitous and persistent. In the 1950s studies concluded that women with CPP showed repressed hostility, anxiety and neuroses, and throughout the 1960s a link was sought for particular psychological characteristics of women with CPP. The advent of laparoscopy in the 1970s allowed doctors to differentiate between those women with definite pathology, such as endometriosis, and those with MUS. It was this latter group that became the focus of attempts to apply psychological labels such as neurosis, sexual dysfunction, depression, and somatization to women with CPP.

The exact link between CPP and sexual abuse is therefore very tenuous, and the mechanism speculative. Studies by their very nature are retrospective and therefore rely on recall, and some are undertaken with small samples. The incidence of sexual abuse of females within the general population is not known with any degree of accuracy, so whether results for women with CPP are significantly different cannot be assessed. More work needs to be carried out prospectively on the long-term experiences of sexual abuse survivors to ascertain whether they suffer more CPP (or other pathology) than the general population, rather than making links retrospectively with the population of women who experience CPP. Without this we may be extrapolating from a link that is present only in a subsection of women, or making causal assumptions from a correlation.

Implications for practice

This chapter has shown that for many women the experience of CPP is unsatisfactory, characterized by many years of pain and by negative encounters with health professionals. This is borne out by much qualitative research on the subject, and recent studies demonstrate very similar findings to those undertaken over a decade ago.

Health professionals can help to improve the experience of women with CPP that remains unexplained in a number of ways, beginning with history taking. 'When the history is taken caringly, with the patient talking and the clinician listening, it establishes rapport. Furthermore, there is great therapeutic benefit from the telling of one's story' (Howard, 2003: 595). Patients need to have their experience believed, and not be labelled on the basis of stereotypes or perceived behaviour. By the time women are seen in a particular setting they may have had many setbacks, and may not therefore behave in a manner that the health professional deems appropriate. It is important for practitioners to consider that depression or weepiness may be the effect of long-term pain rather than a causal mechanism.

Whether or not CPP is associated with sexual abuse, any gynaecological procedure may have a traumatic effect on anyone who has experienced it, provoking flashbacks or reviving memories that had been suppressed. All such procedures need to be undertaken with sensitivity and care to observe any indication of distress. At the same time, we cannot make assumptions about the impact of previous sexual abuse on current pain or on behaviour. Women will deal with it in different ways, and it is important to never assume you know how to interpret an action or behaviour, but to always ask the woman how she is feeling.

In summary, the research cited here has demonstrated that unexplained pain is real pain and health care providers need to avoid making dualistic divisions between visceral and psychosomatic pain, or explained and unexplained pain. Health professionals will frequently reject the patient with

CPP, or collude with them, possibly against another health professional. Neither approach is helpful for the woman in managing her pain. Empowering patients using integrated approaches that present non-biomedical interventions as valuable and worthwhile can offer more treatment choice and is consistent with government policy on patients taking responsibility for and having control over their health.

Summary

Chronic pelvic pain is a common and debilitating gynaecological condition in women which impacts on all aspects of their lives. A diagnosis for the pain is often not achieved, and women may be labelled as having medically unexplained pain. This may carry implications of exaggeration of symptoms, or having the pain psychologized. CPP is also commonly associated with sexual abuse but the evidence on which this is based is tenuous. Women often report negative experiences within the health care system, and may disengage with services if these persist. Health care professionals can improve the experience of women with CPP by listening to their story, and treating them with credibility. Simple dualistic distinctions between types of pain should be avoided. Management of pain needs to be viewed as a positive step, and not as a failure to provide a diagnostic label.

Further reading

Grace, V. and McBride-Stewart, S. (2007) '"Women get this": Gendered meanings of chronic pelvic pain', *Health: An Interdisciplinary Journal for Social Study of Health, Illness and Medicine*, 11(1): 47–67.
Nettleton, S. (2006) '"I just want permission to be ill": Towards a sociology of medically unexplained symptoms', *Social Science and Medicine*, 62: 1167–78.

References

Bendelow, G. (2009) *Health, Emotion and the Body*. Cambridge: Polity Press.
Bendelow, G. and Williams, S. J. (2000) 'Natural for women, abnormal for men. Beliefs about pain and gender', in S. Nettleton and J. Watson (eds), *The Body in Everyday Life*. London: Routledge.
Butler, C.C. and Evans, M. (1999) 'The heartsink patient revisited', *British Journal of General Practice* 49: 230–233.
Denny, E. (2009) '"I never know from one day to another how I will feel" Pain and uncertainty in women with endometriosis', *Qualitative Health Research*, 19(7): 285–95.

Denny, E., Culley, L. and Papadopoulos, I. (2010) *Endometriosis and Cultural Diversity: Improving Services for Minority Ethnic Women. Final Report*. Birmingham: Birmingham City University.

Grace, V. and McBride-Stewart, S. (2007) '"Women get this": Gendered meanings of chronic pelvic pain', *Health: An Interdisciplinary Journal for Social Study of Health, Illness and Medicine*, 11(1): 47–67.

Grace, V. and Zondervan, K. (2006) 'Chronic pelvic pain in women in New Zealand: Comparative well-being, comorbidity, and impact on work and other activities', *Health Care for Women International*, 27: 585–99.

Howard, F.M. (2003) 'Chronic pelvic pain', *Obstetrics and Gynecology*, 101(3): 594–611.

Khan, K.S and Latthe, P. (2009) 'Pelvic pain and ectopic pregnancy', in B. Magowan, P. Owen and J. Drife (eds), *Clinical Obstetrics and Gynaecology*, 2nd edn. Edinburgh: Saunders Elsevier.

Lampe, A., Solder, E., Ennemoser, A., Schubert, C., Rumpold, G. and Sölner, W. (2000) 'Chronic pelvic pain and previous sexual abuse', *Obstetrics and Gynecology*, 96: 929–33.

Latthe, P., Latthe, M., Say, L., Gülmezoglu, M. and Khan, K.S. (2006) 'WHO systematic review of prevalence of chronic pelvic pain: A neglected reproductive health morbidity', *BMC Public Health*, 6: 177. [Online] Available from www.biomedcentral.com/1471-2458/6/177 (accessed 9 August 2010).

McGowan, L., Pitts, M. and Carter, D.C (1999) 'Chronic pelvic pain: The General Practitioner's perspective', *Psychology, Health and Medicine*, 4(3): 303–17.

McGowan, L., Luker, K., Creed, F. and Chew–Graham, C.A. (2007) '"How do you explain a pain that can't be seen?": The narratives of women with chronic pelvic pain and their disengagement with the diagnostic cycle', *British Journal of Health Psychology*, 12: 261–74.

McGowan, L., Escott, D., Luker, K., Creed, F. and Chew-Graham, C. (2010) 'Is chronic pelvic pain a comfortable diagnosis for primary care practitioners: A qualitative study', *BMC Family Practice*, 11: 7. [Online] Available from http://www.biomedcentral.com/1471-2296/11/7 (accessed 13 September 2010).

Nettleton, S. (2006) '"I just want permission to be ill": Towards a sociology of medically unexplained symptoms', *Social Science and Medicine*, 62: 1167–78.

O'Dowd, T. C. (1988) 'Five years of heartsink patients in general practice', *British Medical Journal*, 297: 528–30.

Pitts, M., McGowan, L. and Carter, D. C. (2000) 'Chronic pelvic pain', in J.M. Ussher (ed.), *Women's Health. Contemporary International Perspectives*. Leicester: BPS Books.

Poleshuck, E.L., Dworkin, R.H., Howard, F.M., Foster D.C., Shields, C.G., Giles, D.E. and Tu, X. (2005) 'Contributions of physical and sexual abuse to women's experience of chronic pelvic pain', *Journal of Reproductive Medicine*, 50(5): 91–100.

Randolph, M.E. and Reddy, D. M. (2006) 'Sexual abuse and sexual functioning in a chronic pelvic pain sample', *Journal of Child Sexual Abuse*, 15(3): 61–78.

Rosenburg, C. E. (2002) 'The tyranny of diagnosis: Specific entities and individual experience', *The Milbank Quarterly*, 80(2): 237–60.

Savidge, C.J., Slade, P., Stewart, P. and Li, T.C. (1998) 'Women's perspectives of their experiences of chronic pelvic pain', *Journal of Health Psychology*, 3(1): 103–16.

Sharpe, M. (2001) 'Medically unexplained symptoms and syndromes', *Clinical Medicine*, 2(6): 510–14.

Williams, R.E., Hartmann, K.E. and Steege, J.F. (2004) 'Documenting the current definitions of chronic pelvic pain: Implications for research', *Obstetrics and Gynecology*, 103(4): 686–91

5

Me and ME: Therapeutic Landscapes in an Unfamiliar World

Sara MacKian

Overview

- Living with ME
- An experience of exclusion
- Creating therapeutic landscapes
- Using a spatial framework to understand and support illness experiences

This chapter, based on on-going research, explores the shifting worlds of long-term illness and the emergent landscapes, for people living with ME. There has been previous research on patient's constructions of ME (Guise et al., 2007), and their beliefs about the causes of their condition (Clements et al., 1997), but here I shift the emphasis and focus not on the construction of ME itself, but on the construction of the worlds people live in when living with ME. The landscapes that individuals experience, either physically or mentally, have a profound influence on their overall health and well-being (Williams, 1998: 1199), and there is therefore merit in exploring them as a possible means of developing supportive care environments for those living with long-term debilitating conditions.

A diagnosis of exclusion

A core feature of the world as experienced through ME is exclusion – exclusion from mainstream medicine, exclusion from social worlds, exclusion from one's own sense of self-identity. One reason for such exclusion is a lack of clarity over diagnosis. Early recognized outbreaks during the first half of the twentieth century were often seen as the result of mass hysteria, neurosis and imitated behaviour, and took on the name of their location, for example Royal Free Disease (Chaitow, 1989).

During the late 1980s there emerged a host of labels such as 'yuppie 'flu' (de Wolfe, 2009) or 'closet AIDS' (Chaitow, 1989), but also attempts at pinpointing a name linked to pathology, such as Chronic Fatigue Syndrome (CFS) or Myalgic Encephalomyelitis (ME). Debate continues as to a suitable label for this condition, to such an extent that it has been labelled 'the disease of a thousand names' (Pinching and Freedman, 2003: 80). The label 'ME' has since been shown to be medically inaccurate; however, it has been noted that patients themselves often prefer this name (Guise et al., 2007), as do most of the people I interview. It is also reflected in the two major support organizations in the UK using this name: the ME Association and Action for ME, and this is the label I have chosen to use.

The very nature of ME, with its broad range of symptoms and uneasy diagnosis leads it to be confused with other disorders. Someone with ME may be considered to be suffering from multiple sclerosis, polio, arthritis or depression, which must be first excluded, so that:

> the emphasis on exclusions rather than inclusions tends to characterise the condition as a whole. (Banks and Prior, 2001: 12)

ME is therefore a controversial and problematic illness for all (Guise et al., 2007), and despite the publication of guidance for GPs on ME, confidence with making a diagnosis and managing the condition is low (Bowen et al., 2005), with many in the medical profession refusing to acknowledge its validity. The use of antidepressants remains one of the most commonly offered treatments to those who seek conventional medical help, despite lack of clinical evidence of their efficacy (Lewith, 2002), and there remains a lack of clear research evidence in terms of what works and what does not. This often results in difficult relationships between patients and their care providers (Arroll and Senior, 2008), with patients' ideas frequently conflicting with those of medical practitioners (Horton-Salway, 2004). Even post-diagnosis by a doctor who 'believes in ME', patients have reported a lack of understanding and advice from the medical profession (Edwards et al., 2007). It is an illness you have to fight to get (Dumit, 2006), and one that leaves you in unknown territory in more ways than one.

Journeys to the world of legitimate illness

As the patient embarks on a long and arduous journey to diagnosis, they may begin to struggle in their attempts to uphold normal everyday duties, perhaps having increasing amounts of time off work and failing to find sympathy and support because the doctors cannot find anything 'wrong'. For most journeys into illness, society has a tried and tested model for responding, neatly summarized by American sociologist Talcott Parsons (see box below).

Parson's sick role (Parsons, 1951)

Being labelled legitimately 'sick', the individual enters a period of sanctioned deviance. They are failing to meet the normal obligations of being a productive member of society, but within this temporary identity of 'sick' this is acceptable. They have certain obligations and rights:

Obligations:

- They should try to get well
- They should seek help from, and co-operate with the medical professional

Rights:

- They are exempt from normal social roles
- They are not held responsible for their condition

Parsons' 'sick role' model has not been without its critics (see, for example, Emke, 2002; Fahy and Smith, 1999). However, it does have considerable merit in terms of understanding why people with ME in particular should struggle so much to get their illness validated, professionally and socially. They fail to fulfil the obligations set out in the model, so they cannot benefit from the rights. They are often considered to be 'malingering', or not 'wanting' to get well. Many people with ME have to fight to find a doctor who will diagnose or treat them, so they fail to 'co-operate' with medical professionals. The individual is seen as responsible for bringing this on themselves, and are told it is 'all in the mind' (Hodgkinson, 1988), so they are expected to get on with normal social roles. They are left in a kind of limbo world, no longer in the world of the healthy, yet barred from the world of the sick.

This delayed or blocked entry into a legitimate sick role can aggravate the disease and cause irreparable damage to people's lives as they become increasingly isolated (Edwards et al., 2007). As one of my research participants told me:

> 'you feel very isolated with it ... I mean most illnesses you're just expected to get better. Either you die or you get better after a few months, and you don't with ME that's what's so difficult about it.' (Mandy) (pseudonyms are used for all research participants)

Even once a diagnosis has been reached, some continue to face stigma and disbelief from medical carers (Åsbring and Närvänen, 2002), or family and friends (Edwards et al., 2007). For Mark the uncertainty concerning his illness was too much for his wife to cope with and she left him:

> 'When you get married, it's for better, for worse, you know. Say if my wife had been ill I would've stood by her ... it's just because it's one of those illnesses that's not recognized.'

Hence it is often through a long and painful, frequently tiring and expensive, journey of negative test results and failed prescriptions that an individual arrives at the signpost 'ME'. They have reached a diagnosis through exclusion which points them forwards into a territory of the unknown:

> the path towards a diagnosis of CFS/ME may not have delivered the resolution that had been hoped for. (Arroll and Senior, 2008: 454)

Like many complex syndromes afflicting modern Western society, ME therefore challenges the single, linear trajectory of living with a long-term condition, and the notion that an individual might journey through it according to some available route-map. The metaphor of the linear journey lacks credibility with the ME experience. Not only because patients, like Mandy, are unlikely to know precisely where that journey is going or how long it will take, but also because there are no clearly signposted 'end points' that they are heading for – there are as yet no clear signposts for treatment and prognosis for people living with ME. My research with people with ME has prompted an exploration therefore not of the 'journeys' people are taking *through* this illness, but of the 'landscapes' they live *within* whilst experiencing it.

New worlds, changing worlds

> 'I wanted to do something, people would say, well maybe you shouldn't in case it's too much for you, I just wanted to *scream,* and say but I *want* to do it you know! Let me.' (Liz)

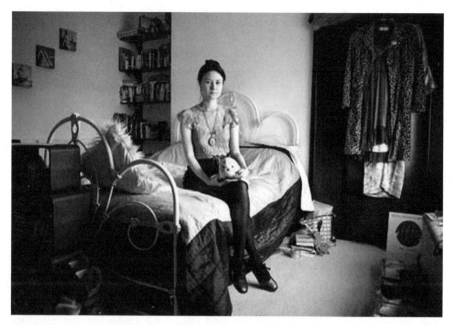

Figure 5.1 'Lucy's Kingdom' (from Chenery-Robson, 2010: 13)

Life with ME can become very static, circumscribed, restricted and one dimensional. These restricted worlds of confinement, alienation, social exclusion and loss of identity are portrayed vividly by Juliet Chenery-Robson in her challenging photographic images (Chenery-Robson, 2010). She portrays the subjects of her images as trapped in the 'Kingdoms of the sick', looking out in a way that challenges the viewer's notions of what living with this condition means in terms of everyday life experience (Figure 5.1).

Chenery-Robson's images powerfully depict the spatial confinement of living with ME. But what lies beyond the room and beyond the embodied presence of the individual? The broader context within which people living with ME find themselves is integral to understanding and locating their stories, and those stories expand beyond the physical confines we might see them in. As Chenery-Robson's images show, they may find themselves 'in' a physically restricted world, but there is more to 'being' in the world than simply where we are located. As Heidegger's concept *Dasein* shows, this is not a simple physical placement:

> If a thing is said to be 'in' something else, this relationship is 'spatial'. If a being of the kind of Dasein is said to be 'in' something, the relationship is not meant to be primarily 'spatial', but means to 'dwell', to 'sojourn', to 'stay'… e.g. a match is in a box in the plain spatial sense; but if a man is in his home or in his office or in a seaside-resort, obviously this relationship is not primarily spatial. (Werner Brock, 1949: 42)

'Being-in-the-world' is fundamentally different to something that is simply 'in' that world, and this suggests the possibility of numerous 'places' occupying one 'space'. We can quite conceivably be perceiving different spaces and places whilst ostensibly inhabiting the same ones. The world can be a very different place for different people. To understand living with ME we need to move beyond describing matches in boxes, to understanding embodied experiences at the seaside.

To build on Werner Brock's seaside analogy, we do not have to be physically 'at' the seaside to relive its atmosphere and therapeutic benefits. Indeed one ME support group held an imaginary day trip to the seaside from the comfort of sufferers' own homes, providing fun and a sense of inclusion manageable even for those house-bound (Williams, 2004). Participants were encouraged to 'bring' sunglasses, buckets and spades, to join in this shared trip to the seaside. A novel and fun idea, but one rooted in an understanding of the value of locating therapeutic moments within the confines of the everyday world.

The impact of our relationship with the social, physical and emotional environment on people's health and well-being has spawned a growing literature on 'therapeutic landscapes' (Smyth, 2005). Therapeutic landscape refers to the physical, social and psychological environment which can be associated with health or well-being (Gesler, 1992). Whilst much of this literature focuses on specific physical locations a person might 'go to' in order to soak up its healing properties (see, for example, Williams, 2010), a therapeutic landscape can also be a discursive space which is constructed and experienced as being conducive to health and well-being (MacKian, 2008).

One of the main reasons respondents in studies of illness say they initially realize something is 'wrong', is because they find they can no longer conduct their lives 'as normal'. They are having to *withdraw* from one or more areas with which they would usually engage, be this in a physical or a social sense. Later on people start to look for new avenues of support or help, and thereby *extend* both their physical and social spatialities. Given this spatial metaphor, it is no wonder then that the idea of therapeutic landscapes has been suggested as a useful one when working in a therapeutic or caring situation to try and help people come to terms with the complex landscape of long-term illness (Williams, 1998).

Worlds within worlds: Creating therapeutic landscapes

An important point to stress, one that is fundamental to the experience of ME in particular, is that there does not have to be physical presence in these therapeutic landscapes. Having a link to the physical world does not necessitate 'going there'. The Chair of a local support group explains:

> 'The most important single thing that we do for members is the newsletter, … some of them are bed bound … they can't get out, so I think the newsletter is the most important thing.' (Derric)

Kate, having attended one meeting of a local ME support group, decided that physical involvement with the group was not for her, but she did feel reassured by knowing they were there:

> 'I just needed the reassurance, you know. I mean I wouldn't really want to get involved that deeply … it was nice just to have them there.'

A subjective or psychological escape from a circumscribed lifeworld has been reported as beneficial in other studies of living with ME. For example, in Reynolds et al.'s (2008) study of women's use of art and craft, one of their respondents said:

> '[W]hen I'm doing my art, I'm out there, I'm at the top of the hill or I'm down by the lake or I'm way, way away in Africa.' (quoted in Reynolds et al., 2008: 1285)

Therapeutic movement

The confusion and helplessness which arises from experiencing ME is extremely disruptive for everyday life, and the individual has to reorder the familiar landmarks in their worlds alongside strange new ones in order to create a landscape which is therapeutic for them. The focus of the world may shift, the pace of life may alter, and the individual's life-path might be redirected. By looking at the way in which an individual engages or disengages with the world around them, it is possible to see the 'movement' within their world. This refers not only to movement between places – such as doctors, support groups and home – but also in terms of the general dynamics of the world they live in. For some there are clear areas of activity – which may involve either a movement through time, or a movement around a particular interest at that time.

For example Mark, whose wife left him because of his ME, found his values altered radically and he put his illness partly down to his previously stressful life. Once he let go of all the stress (work, wife, mortgage) he began to concentrate on getting himself better and appreciating life. This opened up a range of new spaces for him, including support groups, alternative therapies and yoga classes. This reflected itself in a very distinct world of active management at the centre of his world and all previous stressors were placed beyond it, at the boundary. He 'doesn't go there' either physically or subjectively. Mark's world projects into the future, where he envisages health and a new career, and his sphere of active management rolls steadily along that trajectory.

Of course everyone's world is different. Derric has no such time dimension in his world. The central focus of his world is a battle to get ME recognized, to help him regain control over his restricted life, and this is where he directs his activity:

> 'I wrote to about 17 MPs and ministries last year … pointing out that they were spending in the region of 220 million pounds a year in benefits for ME sufferers but virtually nothing on research … You know in this country you can write, I've got a file of letters … It's done a little bit of good I think, but not an awful lot …'

Thus Derric's world is dominated by this advancing battle, advancing not forwards in time but forwards to a place of official recognition.

The dynamics of a therapeutic landscape were clearly very different for Mark and Derric. For Mark a focus on the future gave his world a sense of movement to a future away from ME; for Derric the emphasis was on broader recognition for ME, rather than personally moving beyond it at this time.

Therapeutic 'otherworlds'

Both Mark and Derric had a clear focus in their world which would be easily visible and recognized by others. However, it is not always so obvious to see what features strongly in the world of an individual we do not personally know. Experiencing long-term illness can push people into areas they may not previously have engaged with, that may sit uncomfortably alongside more mainstream approaches. Monica was treated homeopathically for her ME, but is not always forthcoming about this:

> 'I'm very careful who I mention the ME to, and even more careful who I mention the homeopathy to. It worked for me, and I still swear by it, but not all doctors do. You can do it alongside without them having to know anyway!'

ME patients frequently turn to alternative therapies (see, for example, Edwards et al., 2007; Reynolds et al., 2008) so Monica is not alone. Patients are often advised to discuss any alternative therapies with their doctor, but for Monica it appeared more therapeutic *not* to do so. She also found it difficult to discuss her growing spiritual interests with her doctor, but it was something she felt a need to do:

> 'It was really important to me. But I felt a bit daft going in there and talking about it, I didn't want her to think I was mad! But it's helped me come to terms with the ME, it made me realise I've learnt something from this … so there was a reason I got it … She must've picked up on it, because one day she asked about why I thought I had got ME, and it allowed me to at least say I don't know, but I think I've learnt to grow from it and she was good with that, she could see it helped me.'

Monica skirted around the issue of her growing spiritual world, but nonetheless was able to give her doctor a glimpse of this part of her therapeutic landscape that was important for her.

Jess also described to me her experience of engaging with a new spiritual world as a result of ME, when she started attending her local Spiritualist Church for healing:

> 'someone actually spent 20 minutes working exclusively with me … which made me feel valued as an individual again. I went regularly to healing for about 4 years … I'm not able to get along to healing services these days as I've stopped driving and it isn't fair on my husband to have to take me out as soon as he gets in from a long day at work so I get absent healing instead'.

Jess felt similarly to Monica that her spirituality was an important part of her ME, but when asked if she had talked with her GP about her healing:

> 'NO! … Despite that he and I get on well together … I have never discussed spiritual healing with him … I just feel that if it was put on an official form by the GP … I would be considered crazy and I don't see why I should have that said about me when folk that practice other religions would possibly be respected for their beliefs and the comfort they derive from that.'

The author Francesca Brown, during physical confinement brought on by ME, found her experiential world opening up and expanding in unexpected ways when she began seeing and communicating with angels. The huge success of Francesca Brown's subsequent book, *My Whispering Angels* (Brown, 2009), and the growing popularity of other authors with similar experiences of angelic or spiritual aid in recovery from long-term conditions (such as Lorna Byrne's (2009) *Angels in My Hair*), suggest such dimensions to patients' worlds should be acknowledged as legitimate and vital parts of their therapeutic landscapes, even if others may not consider them valid. For some this spiritual link will be a physical engagement, through hands on healing or visiting church. Alternatively it might provide a subjective sense of connection with the physical world, for example through distance healing, or with an otherworld entirely.

Discussion: Back down to earth

[E]ffective treatment requires the doctor to work with patients' descriptions of their experiences rather than imposing their own. (Guise et al., 2007: 105)

Some common treatments for ME are based on precisely the kinds of assumptions that patients themselves reject. For example, many sufferers appear to feel insulted by the offer of support such as CBT (cognitive behaviour therapy), because they infer this to mean 'it is all in the head', even though that may not be the intention when it is offered (Lewith, 2002: 36). For professionals working to support ME sufferers therefore there should be a greater concern with the individual's personal perception of the world rather than the professional's interpretation of the 'reality' of the condition. How people structure their world in response to the experience of ME therefore has important implications for practice, and the features that create a therapeutic landscape will differ in subtle ways for different people. What we can gain by exploring people's experiences within the framework of therapeutic landscapes is an understanding of the dynamics of their worlds. These worlds have been carefully constructed by each individual to help them live with ME. An understanding of this can facilitate better communication with and support from carers, both formal and informal, because it will enable the carer to work within the landscape that works for that individual at that time.

People living with ME find themselves charting new, unfamiliar and often lonely territories. Any kind of understanding of living in those places can surely only benefit the management of such conditions. Inevitably people living with ME will find they have reduced opportunities for everyday social interactions, sometimes even finding themselves excluded from the very groups and services established to give them support, such as ME support groups, either because they are too ill to attend or because they do not like joining such groups (Guise et al., 2007). It is vital therefore to understand the therapeutic value of alternative 'worlds' and how positive support and professional guidance might help individuals construct and manage a therapeutic landscape that serves their needs.

Expanding engagement by introducing new features to a person's therapeutic landscape can, for some, improve self-image and self-confidence through providing meaningful experiences within circumscribed lifeworlds (Reynolds et al., 2008). But this does not have to come in pre-prescribed ways, as the therapeutic landscapes that we might like to see coming out of care relationships are context dependent and variable between individuals. Given the growing popularity of virtual communication and electronic social networks, it might be possible to develop tailored online support environments for individuals which are sympathetic to their lived experience. This would look very different for Derric compared to Mark, for example, whilst Monica and Jess might find their landscapes looked very similar.

Conclusion

> Given that CFS/ME remains an illness with no cure, exploring how people can be helped to cope with the illness is vital for clinicians, sufferers and carers. (Edwards et al., 2007; 210)

Managing long-term conditions is always difficult. Len Sperry, an experienced counsellor, stresses the importance of understanding typical journeys or phases that patients with chronic illness experience, in order to work effectively with them (Sperry, 2009). Seeing long-term conditions through such a phased model is a common approach (Fennell, 2003). I would suggest that it is also helpful to understand that some may not be on such obvious 'journeys' or in clear cut 'phases'. They may be in particular 'places' or 'landscapes' which are equally important to understand.

Co-producing an understanding of the world as experienced by the individual, may be one way of helping professionals, carers, family and friends to live with the individual *in* their world rather than constantly at a distance. This can help to provide the sort of holistic, responsive and contextual care espoused by David Colin-Thomé, the National Director for Primary Care. This chapter has used the idea of therapeutic landscapes as one way of achieving this, a concept also popular amongst psychologists, counsellors and clinicians (Williams, 1998). However, it should be remembered that places are not 'intrinsically therapeutic', but will be experienced in different ways by different people (Conradson, 2005). What is experienced as healing for one person will be perceived as inherently damaging by another. Not everyone would have wanted to join the day trip to the seaside. The healing properties of any particular feature in a person's therapeutic landscape must therefore be defined by and understood from that individual's perspective, in order for any carer to work effectively with them (Williams, 1998).

Respondents in research often report a general lack of professional advice about living positively with ME (Reynolds et al., 2008).

> Many health care professionals are caught in a tradition of 'rehabilitating' people with chronic illness by assisting them to accept the limitations imposed by their disease. Such an approach may be counterproductive. For example, losses and limitations may not be viewed negatively by a person with chronic illness but rather as opportunities for transformation. (Paterson, 2001: 25)

Indeed, 'losses and limitations' may translate into gains and expansion. Whilst I do not wish to suggest every experience of ME can allow the individual to open up new and exciting worlds of experience, I do want to stress that the possibility is there, and this should be acknowledged. For those who do not experience such positive transformations, a better understanding of what their world looks like for them can help to provide appropriate and sensitive support and care.

ME no longer hits the headlines in the same way as it did in the 1980s and 1990s, though it remains prevalent and controversial (de Wolfe, 2009), and frequently 'overwhelming and isolating' (Edwards et al., 2007: 210). Medical science has yet to find any solutions or magic fixes. Perhaps then, one constructive way we can move forward is to use social science to understand the situated experience of living with ME, and support each individual to live in harmony with their particular world.

Summary

Experiencing long-term illness alters the everyday world. Using a spatial metaphor and the notion of therapeutic landscapes reveals how individuals restructure their everyday worlds of experience to cope with their changing circumstances. Understanding of this could be usefully developed when caring for or managing long-term conditions.

Acknowledgements

I would like to thank Juliet Chenery-Robson for kindly allowing me to reproduce 'Lucy's Kingdom', and wish her continued success with her photographic projects which so successfully and powerfully visualize the invisible illness ME.

Further reading

MacKian, S. (2000) 'Contours of coping: Mapping the subject world of long-term illness', *Health and Place*, 6: 95–104.

MacKian, S. (2004) 'Mapping reflexive communities: Visualising the geographies of emotion', *Journal of Social and Cultural Geography*, 5(4): 615–31.

http://www.afme.org.uk/

http://www.meassociation.org.uk/

References

Arroll, M.A. and Senior, V. (2008) 'Individuals' experience of chronic fatigue syndrome/myalgic encephalomyelitis', *Psychology and Health*, 23(4): 443–58.

Åsbring, P. and Närvänen, A.-L. (2002) 'Women's experiences of stigma in relation to chronic fatigue syndrome and fybromyalgia', *Qualitative Health Research*, 12: 148–60.

Banks, J. and Prior, L. (2001) 'Doing things with illness: The micro politics of the CFS clinic', *Social Science and Medicine*, 52: 11–23.

Bowen, J., Pheby, D., Charlett, A. and McNulty, C. (2005) 'Chronic fatigue syndrome: A survey of GPs' attitudes and knowledge', *Family Practice: An International Journal*, April: 389–93.

Brown, F. (2009) *My Whispering Angels*. London: Hodder and Stoughton.

Byrne, L. (2009) *Angels In My Hair*. London: Arrow Books.

Chaitow, L. (1989) *Post-viral Fatigue Syndrome*. London: JM Dent and Sons Ltd.

Chenery-Robson, J. (2010) *A Diagnosis of Exclusion* [Online]. Available at Blurb.com

Clements, A., Sharpe, M., Simkin, S. and Borrill, J. (1997) 'Chronic fatigue syndrome: A qualitative investigation of patients' beliefs about the illness', *Journal of Psychosomatic Research*, 42: 615–24.

Conradson, D. (2005) 'Landscape, care and the relational self', *Health and Place*, 11: 337–48.

De Wolfe, P. (2009) 'ME: The rise and fall of a media sensation', *Medical Sociology Online*, 4(1): 2–13.

Dumit, J. (2006) 'Illnesses you have to fight to get', *Social Science and Medicine*, 62(3): 577–90.

Edwards, C.R., Thompson, A.R. and Blair, A. (2007) 'An "overwhelming illness": Women's experiences of learning to live with chronic fatigue syndrome/myalgic encephalomyelitis', *Journal of Health Psychology*, 12(2): 203–14.

Emke, I. (2002) 'Patients in the New Economy: The "sick role" in a time of economic discipline', *Animus*, 7: 81–93.

Fahy, K. and Smith, P. (1999) 'From the sick role to subject positions: A new approach to the medical encounter', *Health*, 3(1): 71–94.

Fennell, P. (2003) *Managing Chronic Illness: The Four Phase Approach*. New York: John Wiley.

Gesler, W. (1992) 'Therapeutic landscapes: Medical issues in light of the new cultural geography', *Social Science and Medicine*, 34(7): 735–46.

Guise, J., Widdicombe, S. and McKinlay, A. (2007) '"What is it like to have ME": The discursive construction of ME in computer-mediated communication and face-to-face interaction', *Health,* 11(1): 87–108.

Hodgkinson, N. (1988) '"Yuppie flu" is all in the mind, say doctors', *Sunday Times,* 17 July.

Horton-Salway, M. (2004) 'The local production of knowledge: Disease labels, identities and category entitlements in ME support group talk', *Health,* 8(3): 351–71.

Lewith, G. (2002) 'Research update: Examining the alternative', *InterAction,* 42: 35–7.

MacKian, S. (2008) 'What the papers say: Reading therapeutic landscapes of women's health and empowerment in Uganda', *Health and Place,* 14(1): 106–15.

Parsons, T. (1951) *The Social System.* London: Routledge and Kegan Paul.

Paterson, B. (2001) 'The shifting perspectives model of chronic illness', *Journal of Nursing Scholarship,* First Quarter: 21–6.

Pinching, A. and Freedman, L. (2003) 'AIDS and CFS/ME: A tale of two syndromes', *Clinical Medicine,* 3(1): 78–82.

Reynolds, F., Vivat, B. and Prior, S. (2008) 'Women's experiences of increasing subjective well-being in CFS/ME through leisure-based arts and crafts activities: A qualitative study', *Disability and Rehabilitation,* 30(17): 1279–88.

Smyth, F. (2005) 'Medical geography: Therapeutic places, spaces and networks', *Progress in Human Geography,* 29(4): 488–95.

Sperry, L. (2009) 'Therapeutic response to patients and families experiencing chronic medical conditions', *The Family Journal,* 17 (April): 180–4.

Werner Brock, P. (1949) 'An account of "Being and Time"', in M. Heidegger (ed.), *Existence and Being.* London: Vision Press. pp. 25–248.

Williams, A. (1998) 'Therapeutic landscapes in holistic medicine', *Social Science and Medicine,* 46(9): 1193–203.

Williams, A. (2010) 'Spiritual therapeutic landscapes and healing: A case study of St. Anne de Beaupre, Quebec, Canada', *Social Science and Medicine,* 70(10): 1633–40.

Williams, Z. (2004) 'Still live', *InterAction,* 49: 22–3.

WORKING WITH PEOPLE WITH LONG-TERM CONDITIONS

Introduction

Tom Heller

This section contains five chapters that consider various aspects of working with people with long-term conditions from very different viewpoints. Because the authors approach the subject area from different directions the totality of the section covers many of the most important aspects of this topic.

The first chapter in this section, 'How to Make Health and Social Care Research Radical and Really, Really Useful', looks at the way that people with long-term conditions can and should be involved in research that deals with the issues that are central to their lives. The chapter is presented in the form of a heart-felt debate between the two authors: Rachel Purtell, who is a long-term user of health and social care services, and Andy Gibson, an experienced researcher and academic. The debate is conducted in a warm, friendly and self-disclosing manner, but uncovers many of the complexities and practical difficulties that researchers continue to experience in their attempts to include people who use health and social care services in research in a meaningful way. Rachel, in her turn, is clear that much research that purports to include people with long-term conditions who use health and social care services can turn out to be tokenistic, patronizing and full of practical hurdles to be overcome. Andy remains optimistic that some of the problems of involving people who use health and social care services in research can be overcome by a mixture of allocating a realistic amount of resources, clear policy directives and flexibility by all parties. The message remains though that 'really really' including people with long-term conditions in the research that will affect their lives is a special skill that requires new ways of working – but that without this effort the research will always be of limited usefulness.

The following chapter by Tom Heller, 'Naught for Your Comfort: Quality of Primary Care for People with Long-term Conditions', takes a case history approach that looks at a 60-year old person who suddenly develops a long-term condition. 'Eric' has a stroke that immediately propels him into being a person with needs. The transition puts a strain on Eric, his self-image and his family relationships. Health and social care services are found to be lacking, in particular the lack of co-ordination between services causes additional problems ensuring that Eric and others like him fall between the gaps. Deficiencies in service provision for people with long-term conditions have been exposed by research and official surveys, but despite well meaning official policy statements, the actual experience for people like Eric remains patchy and unpredictable. New ways of working in health and social services seem to focus on 'efficiency', often seemingly at the expense of continuity and even humanity. The reward system within primary care that provides payment for the teams of health care professionals looking after people with long-term conditions such as stroke seems to reward clinical and formulaic care at the expense (literally) of more person-centred types of caring. The introduction of 'payment by results' for primary care teams has led to instances of 'gaming' and manipulation of those results in order to maximize payment – but with no evidence of improvement in the quality of care experienced by people who use the services or their carers.

Chapter 8, 'Diabetes and Pregnancy: Service-users' Perspectives on Services and on Research', by Cathy E. Lloyd and Sarah Earle, is based on qualitative research that looked in detail at a group of women who were both pregnant and had diabetes. These two conditions separately pose searching questions for health and social care services as well as for all professional practitioners in those services – but the combination of conditions adds additional complexity and a series of new challenges. Both conditions are potentially risky in terms of possible complications and recent policy directives seem focused on the prevention of tangible clinical problems – but at the expense of attention to the perceived needs and psychosocial requirements of women living with the reality of both conditions. The particular concern of people from different ethnic backgrounds emerges clearly from these stories. Many women felt that their need for support and reassurance had not been met while the staff attended to, and became almost fixated by, clinical issues such as blood sugar measurement and control. Indeed access to 'normal' types of care, for example by community midwives, was not routinely available because women with diabetes and pregnancy were deemed to need specialist services that may not include more general supportive types of pregnancy care. Research into these conditions has traditionally been *performed on* the women with these two conditions. But this chapter describes the way that women with the experience of diabetes during pregnancy are keen to help to mould further research, the outcome of which will be valuable for the future design of services.

Chapter 9, 'Coeliac Disease: Psychosocial Factors in Adults and Children', explores the available literature from both sides of the Atlantic that has looked in great detail into the experience of living with coeliac disease. In this chapter Ruth Howard and her co-authors document the struggle that adults and children with this long-term condition have to lead a normal life, with reference to a large number of published qualitative and quantitative research studies. Because the disease may not have any external manifestations it is often diagnosed only after a long delay during which time people with the condition may be feeling poorly, often in non-specific ways. Even after diagnosis the need to stick to a strict diet without gluten sets them apart from other members of their family and their social groups. A picture emerges of the life of restriction and 'otherness' that children and adults with coeliac disease go through and the possible problems that this can create. Feeling different and possibly excluded while growing up may result in a range of emotional symptoms and a generally lower quality of life than their peers. The parents and carers of young people with coeliac disease often describe a feeling of burden that comes with the additional work involved in arranging a gluten-free diet at all times. For adults with coeliac disease the condition can lead to anger, sadness and pervading tiredness. Always being aware of the need for 'special' dietary arrangements and the curbing of spontaneity creates difficulties in the social arena. However a message of hope emerges; when people, young or older, become stabilized and receive suitable support services the condition can be successfully controlled and any psychosocial manifestations minimized or overcome.

The final chapter in this section of the book by Mary Larkin, 'Working with Vulnerable People: Experiences of Disability', espouses the social model of disability and considers the way that services and practitioners could and should work within this model. Mary Larkin argues that a lot of adjustment to policies and services is needed because of the dominance of the medical model and the potentially damaging effect that this has on the lives of people living with impairment. The social model of disability throws light on the myriad ways that contemporary society creates disability and inequality by discrimination, social oppression and inaccessibility of the built environment. Although recent legislation and official policy pronouncements move the agenda in a progressive direction many services have failed to live up to the standards that have been set by the best services – to the detriment of many people who are not able bodied. The chapter does provide an indication of some of the positive ways that progressive policy can be translated into improvement in the lives of people who previously were passive recipients of services. Personal budgets, direct payments and the entire personalization agenda is discussed and a case study describes the way that more positive outcomes can be achieved. Individual health and social care workers are exhorted to take note of the new policy imperatives and use them imaginatively to improve the lives of people who are currently disadvantaged because of their impairments.

6

How to Make Health and Social Care Research Radical and Really, Really Useful

Rachel Purtell and Andy Gibson

Overview

- How can people with long-term conditions and other users of health and social services really be involved in relevant research?
- In what practical, ethical and principled ways can people make a meaningful contribution to, and have real influence on, research activities that may affect their lives?
- Redistribution of power will be required if people who use services are to become the main driver in the research process and not simply research subjects

Christmas time 2000, the millennium was dawning, but I was celebrating quite a different milestone. On the 18 December 2000 I, yes me – who had been advised to work as a volunteer for the Samaritans by a careers officer at my 'special school', whose educational achievements were somewhat dismal for a whole host of reasons, not least because of the barriers that disabled people face in education and the system's difficulty in coping with people like me – graduated at the University of Leeds with a Master of Arts in Disability Studies. It had possibly been the hardest two years of my life. True, the Snowdon Awards had funded my place on the course, but I had also worked full time while studying the distance learning course.

On the same day I graduated I was handed a job advert by my Professor, Colin Barnes, the man who had also put his money where his mouth is and accepted me on the course in the first place (for which I will be eternally grateful). The advert was for a Research Fellow at the University of Exeter, to co-ordinate the Folk.us Programme. Folk.us was, and is, an organization funded by the National Institute for Health Research (NIHR), which aims to bring the world of researchers and service users closer together.

A month later I was working out how to get myself moved to Exeter and thinking how utterly bizarre life can be! I was about to start work in a University, me of all people, with my solid working class roots, having had in excess of 80 bone fractures as well as being dyslexic and hearing impaired. Me, who when asked what support I needed, said, 'Well I really won't know until I get there!'.

Folk.us, what a job, what a way to make a living! I even get to interview people for jobs, people like my friend here, Andy Gibson.

Andy: I first met Rachel in March 2009. She was on the interview panel for my current job as a Research Fellow in Patient and Public Involvement (I'll explain what that means a bit later on). To be honest I didn't think I was going to get the job, but I did, and a little over three months later I, and my family, were heading from the Midlands to a new life in Devon. Funny where you end up – I left school at 16 with a handful of GCSEs. My first job was as a fitter with what was then known as the National Coal Board. It was bad timing. I started work in 1982, just two years before the miner's strike began. Anyway we lost the strike and in 1989 I was made redundant. I'd been doing some 'O' and 'A' levels in the evening at the local FE college and so I decided to apply for a place at university and managed to get in. So began a journey that brought me to the Peninsula Medical School via a route that included a few years as a social worker and doing a PhD with the Open University. Anyway here I was feeling a bit pleased with myself – and a bit nervous about all the things I said I could do at the interview and which I would now be expected to prove that I could! I'd drifted into the area of service user involvement in research while in a previous job at Warwick University. I'd enjoyed this part of the work and I'd learnt that I'd got some of the necessary skills – such as being able to talk to different audiences and all kinds of people. Perhaps my peculiar career route made it easier for me to have one foot in academia and another in the 'real world', whatever that means. Perhaps this would be a good point to explain what service user involvement, or patient and public involvement (PPI), is. Here we run into our first problem. Although lots of people use these words (in fact it's become very fashionable), it's not altogether clear that we are all talking about the same thing. This can lead to some odd experiences particularly when you realize, part way through a meeting, that you and some of the others in the room share very little in the way of a common understanding of PPI, beyond knowing what the initials stand for.

Rachel: Welcome to my world Andy! See, the thing is that PPI isn't a term we tend to use in Folk.us, we have always stuck with 'Service Users' as defined by Viv Lindow and Jenny Morris (1995: 1): 'People who need some kind of support in order to live in the community, (or take part in the community)'. At Folk.us we also use the phrase 'Service users, patients and carers to inform and guide research at all stages' (Folk.us, 2008–9). The debate about language and about how we describe people is a very long and complex one that we could spend this entire chapter on – and still be no nearer any kind of answer. For someone like me, I feel the issue is somewhat clearer on a personal level yet more complicated when relating to the external world. In my own world it is simply a question of my identity at any given time in any given situation. I am someone who is defined as a 'service user', 'patient', 'disabled person', 'someone who has a long-term condition' and 'Research Fellow'. All of these terms can be appropriate. I'm very clear about what I mean when I use the term 'Disabled Person'. I mean the term to be attached to a very clear Social Model of Disability approach (Oliver, 1983). That is I am someone who has a physical impairment, but is disabled by societal structures (from attitudes to physical barriers). This disabling effect is experienced by many disabled people. When I talk about service users, then the definition of Lindow and Morris fits very well, but I'm also referred to as a 'patient', well I'm a pretty heavy user of health care services, and 'patient' is how we are described. However no one really fits exclusively into these categories, just like most peoples' lives.

Andy: Rachel, I think you raise a very important point here. Some of these terms such as 'service user', have been promoted by people who have direct experience of living with an impairment and experience disability and who have campaigned for things like better services. Other terms like 'Patient and Public Involvement', have been thought up by organizations such as the NHS. There is an important difference here between 'top down' and 'bottom up' approaches. I think in terms of involvement in research there are examples of both approaches. There are research projects where the initial ideas have come from service users, and others where the ideas come from clinicians or academics. I think both are needed, but something very important is missed if we don't ensure that there are mechanisms which allow service users to influence the research agenda. This can be via suggesting what questions should be researched, or by ensuring that service users have a say in which research projects it is important to fund.

Rachel: Or by supporting service users, patients or carers to become co-researchers in their own right, Andy. I also think there is a different 'stake' in all of these things. I do think that there are different issues in involvement for people who need health and social services to support their daily lives, as opposed to those who use health services very occasionally. That's not to say that occasional service users, or patients, don't have important things to say, but they are different. At Folk.us we tend to focus on regular service users, patients and the carers, who have a slightly different interest in all this, but are deeply affected by what happens in services.

I always find it somewhat amusing when some dear eminent researcher in academia, expects Folk.us to have a bunch of 'patients' in a warehouse out back. They roll off the list of characteristics they are wanting in the 'patients we want to involve in our research'. At the end when I say, '*so, you wouldn't want someone like me then?*' they turn a strange colour and bluster about a little. Then as I gently take apart their notion of patients that fit in to their box, we move on to the idea that perhaps they need to think what sort of experience it might be important for a patient to bring to their project. Perhaps more importantly what sort of support their project will offer the patient to enable them to be involved. But equally it can work in reverse. On more than one occasion I've been contacted by an academic who has asked, 'Can I add your name as the service user or as the patient representative, to our bid?' I reply, 'What is the bid about?', 'Chest function while running up a mountain'. Me, 'Mmm… and how exactly would I be representative, of who and of what, as clearly I'm not about to run up a mountain?' Yes that is a little extreme, though not as extreme as you might imagine. The whole issue of who fits into what box in involvement is very live. It frustrates me intensely. For years there has been work involving people who use services and research that has been service user led, but sometimes it feels like hardly anyone employed professionally to do 'PPI' has read it! If we were really doing involvement well and properly we would start entirely from the other end. The people we most need as part of the involvement movement are the ones here using the service. At Folk.us we do probably get closer to the idea that people who really do use the services tell us what they want to do. Even when Andy and I speak I sometimes think, 'that's me you're talking about not "a" group, "a" patient or "a" service user – but people like me', though I suspect I might be equally putting the non-service user, non-disabled people, non-long-term patient world into a group – am I Andy?

Andy: I don't think you are. However, one of the first questions to ask is why are people being involved in the first place? Is this based on an ethical commitment that people have a right to be involved, because it might improve the quality of the research or is it about creating some form of democratic accountability? All these things lead to different ways of approaching involvement but the assumptions underlying them are frequently not spelt out. Even when we talk about occasional users of services I think there are important differences in the experience of health and illness and of services. For example, there is research which suggests that doctors share more information with patients they perceive to be better educated (i.e. more like themselves), than they do with other patients (Tuckett et al., 1985). This straight away creates a basic inequality in the treatment that even occasional users of health and social care receive. I hope this is changing. People are less likely to accept what doctors or other professionals say at face value, and they have access to alternative sources of information via things like the internet, albeit of variable quality. This, plus other factors such as advances in medical science that impact on all our lives, means that the pressure for user involvement is likely to increase – although different governments will undoubtedly put their own political spin on it.

However in order to take service user involvement in research seriously it would be necessary to start at the beginning and ask why academics predominately decide what research questions get asked? It should be just as common for service users to be asking the research questions and prioritizing research projects for funding as it is for academics to be involved in these processes. This is something that we both feel strongly about and have worked on to develop. If this happened research would probably be much better at addressing the health needs of service users and would probably save the NHS a bit of cash by spending less money on inappropriate research or badly delivered services.

Another important issue in the world of research is that we slip into using language like 'health impact', 'disease burdens', 'epidemiology of this or that condition', etc. Sometimes it's useful to think in these terms, but all too frequently these words can distance academics and health professionals from the realities of people's lives. This distance, which is sometimes defended on the grounds of objectivity, can frequently result in research which doesn't address the needs and concerns of service users and carers, or which results in new services and treatments that aren't very accessible or easy to use – particularly by those who need them most. I'm all for the highest possible standards in research, but I also think that one of the many important contributions that user involvement can make to health and social care research is ensuring that the needs of people who are supposed to benefit from all of this are at the very centre of the research process. There is more recognition of this now. Many research funding bodies make user involvement a prerequisite for funding, such as the Research for Patient Benefit programme (see NIHR, 2010 website) but I think some academics still treat it in a superficial, patronizing or over-simplistic way, don't you Rachel?

Rachel: Mmmm, well yes! I think mostly they just start in the wrong place all together. Partly I think there is an overwhelming and wrong headed need to control the process on behalf of academia and services. *'Tell people how they will be involved'*; I say *'No, no, no'*. Tell people the parameters you or your project is working in, what resources you have to support the work including their involvement, what timescale you have. But do not limit their role before you even begin, that is simply opposite to the point of having them there at all. Projects and initiatives have limits, but the wealth of people's experience does not.

I and others like me, occupy this strange world; I'm a Research Fellow, disabled person and service user. In many ways I think our presence in this world is a challenge. Andy shall I talk about the amount of 'PPI' events funded in one way or another by the Department of Health that are physically inaccessible to anyone with mobility or hearing impairments, etc? They are designed for non-service users or non-patients, people who seem to be doing 'involvement' for a living, but who are not themselves people who use services. It appears they only apply the value or need for access if they know it's 'for a group of patients' not that it's part of a good value base to work from, or will you?

Andy: Since you ask I will! Sometimes researchers are concerned that going through the motions of 'doing user involvement' can take up a lot of time and money, while adding little to their research. Alternatively they see it only in terms of the benefit it can give to them or their work. This can lead to people 'doing involvement' in a superficial, half-hearted or mechanical way. Unfortunately these examples of bad research practice happen all too frequently. Of course if the process of involvement is done badly it isn't surprising that the benefits are unclear. It would be like carrying out a piece of research badly and then saying, when the results are inevitably inconclusive, 'See, I told you this research was a waste of time.' This kind of experience can be very damaging for both academics and service users and have the precise opposite effect to what is intended. As Brett et al. (2010) point out, the negative effect on service users can be that they feel overburdened, not listened to, frustrated and marginalized. The key issue here is that user involvement is seen as something that is done to people rather than with them. When I see this happening I sometimes feel it would have been better if they hadn't attempted any involvement at all. At least that way they wouldn't have done any damage!

So what should involving people in health and social care research be about? I think it is about giving the people who are meant to benefit from this research a say in shaping all aspects of the research agenda. It requires service users to be involved on the same basis as academics and health care professionals. This includes not just participating in research that has been initiated by academics, but also in shifting the power balance so that users and carers are encouraged to initiate research in which professionals are invited to offer their skill and expertise. The interactions and relationships between researchers and service users should be based on mutual benefit rather than researchers extracting useful knowledge and experience for their own benefit. This is partly based on an ethical principle that service users have a right to influence research priorities. More pragmatically it should ensure that the research deals explicitly with service users' needs and perceptions of the issues – which will increase the probability of effective use of the research in practice. Of course this means ensuring that user involvement becomes as equally integral to health and social care research as good methodology is. Bringing this about in practice would require a fundamental change in how systems operate and a fundamental shift in power.

Rachel: One advantage to being someone like me in this area of work is that often, though not always, I can explain the need for systems to change, not from a distance, but from direct experience. Folk.us tends to work from the idea that what is essential is to create the right conditions which allow involvement to take place. I think the crucial thing to understand in involvement is that if you get the process right, which means all the boring stuff, then you can pretty much let the outcomes take care of themselves. People think the dull stuff, like sorting payment for people, which generally means hours arguing with your finance department, getting car parking right, finding a format for the written material, is about how you get to involvement. It's not! It is a fundamental part of DOING involvement because if you do that stuff it means that you are valuing what people contribute enough to have had that argument with the finance department. I guess this is second nature to me – the idea of creating the right conditions. Certainly this seems time and time again to be what works. Then all you really need to do is give people the space, the subject matter, or the freedom to come up with their own subjects for research. Currently there is too much emphasis on fitting people into a box and setting too many restrictions. However that is not surprising as the fundamental concept of involvement is to hand over control of the issues. I guess the other thing that is difficult is that involvement isn't meant to be comfortable. Although it does need to be safe for the people involved it is also meant to challenge the status quo. Too often involvement is approached as the need to get service users or patients or carers trained so they will all behave in the same way – again this misses the point.

It also gets forgotten that involvement isn't simply about 'letting the issues be raised' it's about finding the solutions together too. The 'so what' is something we need to ask of much research and again we need people deeply involved with working out those answers too.

There is a huge emphasis on measuring the amount of involvement that has taken place in funded research. This makes sense in terms of public expenditure – the public accountability argument – and no one wants to be wasting public funding especially in 2010. However, it is something that service users involved in research need to be cautious about. In the same way that people tend to be fitted into the 'involvement box', there is a danger of trying to fit involvement into a box that can be measured in separate parts. If the research appears to lead to successful outcomes the danger is to say 'that works so if we just repeat it, it will work again'. Good involvement is never like that because it is an organic growing and changing thing, so you can't repeat it; you can attempt to create similar conditions each time, but it will never be the same – nor should it be.

One of the reasons that there are problems with putting effective involvement into health and social care research is that it requires systems that adapt and change; that is the point, involvement is supposed to challenge and change things – including how whole systems run. This is also reflected in the reality of the lives of individuals living with long-term conditions who are involved in research. An example is that, as a member of University staff, I am subject to the HM Revenue and Custom rules on staff expenses. That's fine, except that for dinner (while away on University business) the allowance is £13.50, which is pretty low. Add to that the need to find somewhere at the end of a long working day that has good wheelchair access, that is near to where I'm staying in somewhere like London and you get to see how all these difficulties start to stack up. We will, with the support of my University, write to HM Revenue and Customs to ask if I might be allowed a higher allowance. This is where whole system approaches become important. During my time at Folk.us, both on a personal level and working on behalf of Folk.us, I have always tried to explain what we need from the systems that have been established to support our work. Involvement is never just about the project or piece of work that you are currently focused on, but always requires a whole system approach. We have to be willing to take on a whole range of issues or involvement will only ever be tokenistic. This dull, boring stuff is actually about the day-to-day lives and barriers lots of us face. It is a challenge in itself. It bothers me greatly that the 'bread and butter' of making involvement work will simply be overlooked. Furthermore, if we really believe that what we are doing has merit we should simply see involvement as one of the ingredients in successful health and social care research. We've emphasized in this chapter the importance of embedding PPI in the entire research process so it seems illogical to me to come up with measurement ideas that explicitly separate involvement from the whole project and examine it as a separate entity. I don't think it makes any sense Andy.

Andy: I agree and I think in evaluating user involvement a burden of proof should not be placed on service users that isn't placed on other members of a research team. At the same time I think service users do want to know that they have made a difference to the research. It is important to improve practice in user involvement, but in a way that moves beyond simple 'How to' toolkits to take account of precisely the type of complexity we have been discussing. Joanna Brett and her colleagues (Brett et al., 2010) in a recent literature review on the impact of user involvement emphasize the importance of separating context and process. They define context as whether the right conditions are in place for involvement and process as the specific factors around the way in which involvement is carried out. They suggest that these factors could be described as the 'architecture' of involvement and suggest that if they are not appropriately established the chances of beneficial impact seem to diminish. Any evaluation of the impact of involvement on research needs to take these factors into account. Anyway, perhaps the interaction between aims, processes, context and outcomes is a whole new debate or material for another chapter!

Summary

In this chapter we have attempted to cover some of the issues that arise when trying to ensure that the involvement of people with long-term conditions becomes an integral part of health and social research that may affect their lives. We have jointly authored this chapter in an attempt to clarify the issues for ourselves and for people reading the chapter. In summary we might say that if involvement is worth doing then it is worth doing properly or not at all. Getting all the facets of user involvement in research right involves getting stuck into detail as well as sticking to important underlying principles. Dealing with the 'boring stuff' is important not because someone says you should do it, but because it has a real and profound effect on the lives of people with a long-term condition. We have also tried to show that simple boxes don't work. Rachel went from being a badly educated disabled woman, to Research Fellow, to Folk.us director, and is now generally thought to be very good at what she does.

We have also tried to outline some of the current debates about involvement, the need for evidence about its effectiveness versus the risks of turning involvement into something that fits neatly in a box, which we feel is counter to good involvement.

Acknowledgements

The writing of this chapter was partially supported by funding from the National Institute for Health Research (NIHR). The views expressed in this publication are those of the authors and not necessarily those of the NHS, the NIHR or the Department of Health.

Further reading

AMRC and TwoCan Associates (2010) *User Involvement in Research: A Route Map* [Online]. Available at: http://www.twocanassociates.co.uk/routemap/. This is an interactive route map for health research charities and other organizations that commission research who wish to involve service users in their work.

Barnes, C. (2003) 'What a difference a decade makes: Reflections on doing "emancipatory" disability research', *Disability and Society*, 18(1): 3–17(15).

Beresford, P. (2002) 'User involvement in research and evaluation: Liberation or regulation?', *Social Policy & Society*, 1: 95–105.

INVOLVE website at www.invo.org.uk. Supports public involvement in NHS, public health and social care research.

Minogue, V. and Girdlestone, J. (2009) 'Building capacity for service user and carer involvement in research: The implications and impact of best research', *International Journal of Health Care Quality Assurance*, 23(4): 422–35.

Mitchell, A. and Purtell, R. (2009) 'Community approaches, social inclusion and user involvement', in S. Llewelyn, P. Kennedy and H. Beinart (eds), *Clinical Psychology in Practice*. Oxford: Wiley-Blackwell.

Rickard, W. and Purtell, R. (2011) 'Finding a way to pay in the UK: Methods and mechanisms for paying service users involved in research', *Disability & Society*, 26(1): 33–48.

References

Brett, J. Staniszewska, S., Mockford, C., Seers, K., Herron-Marx, S. and Bayliss, H. (2010) *The PIRICOM Study: A Systematic Review of the Conceptualisation, Measurement, Impact and Outcomes of Patients and Public Involvement in Health and Social Care Research.* UKCRC [Online]. Available at: http://www.ukcrc.org/patientsandpublic/ppi/understandingppi/ (accessed 10 January 2011).

Folk.us *Annual Report* 2008-2009 (available at: www.folkus.org.uk).

Lindow, V. and Morris, J. (1995) *Service User Involvement.* York: Joseph Rowntree Foundation.

National Institute for Health Research (2010) *The Research for Patient Benefit (RfPB) Programme.* [Online]. Available at: http://www.nihr-ccf.org.uk/site/programmes/rfpb/default.cfm (accessed 16 December 2010).

Oliver, M. (1983) *Social Work with Disabled People.* Basingstoke: Macmillan.

Tuckett, D., Boulton, M., Olsen, C. and Williams, A. (1985) *Meetings Between Experts: An Approach to Sharing Ideas in Medical Consultations.* London: Tavistock.

7

Naught for Your Comfort: Quality of Primary Care for People with Long-term Conditions

Tom Heller

Overview

- Transition to being a person with a long-term condition
- Continuity and quality of primary care
- Managerial responses aimed to improve the quality of care for people with stroke within primary care
- Integrated services for people who have had a stroke

Transition to being a person with a long-term condition

Eric was 60 years old, within days of retirement from his job as an electrical contractor, when he had a stroke. The blocked artery in his brain left him unconscious for several days and affected the power throughout the right side of his body. Ever since the stroke he has been unable to speak or propel himself in the wheelchair to which he became confined. Barbara, his wife, was 57 when this event happened. She is self employed and works as a book keeper for several small local firms.

(Continued)

After two months in the nearby hospital Stroke Unit, Eric was discharged quite late on a Friday afternoon. The following Monday morning Barbara came to her general practitioner's surgery with a discharge note from the hospital. She was angry that no arrangements had been made for caring for Eric over the weekend, and that nobody from the practice had bothered to visit them yet. She was unclear what would happen next.

The transition from being an apparently fit and healthy person to becoming someone with a long-term condition can be sudden and feel very harsh. For Eric and Barbara in the story above, their change in status was dramatic and entirely unwelcome. Before Eric's stroke they had planned some holidays together and had bought a new camper van to celebrate his impending retirement.

There may be a number of transitions involved in the care arrangements for people with long-term conditions. In the story about Eric and Barbara there has been the sudden transition from self-care, during the time before Eric's stroke when they looked after their own and each other's needs – to the undisputable need for more formal types of care in secondary and tertiary care (the local hospital and its Stroke Unit). The vignette above describes a later, unsatisfactory transition from hospital-based care to primary care. Each of these transitions brings uncertainty, anxiety and a complex set of unanswered questions. Often these relate to questions of responsibility. Whose responsibility will it be to look after Eric? How will this responsibility be negotiated between the different parties involved in Eric's future care? Good quality care for people with long-term conditions almost always involves complicated practical arrangements as well as particular attention to detail at these times of transition.

Although the experience of having a stroke might feel to the individual as though it is a random event, in fact there are definite patterns of stroke within communities throughout the UK. The experience of having a stroke is not equally distributed throughout society. Death rates from stroke are three times higher in some poorer areas of the UK than in more affluent areas; 29 deaths per 100,000 men aged under 65 each year in the poorest areas compared with just 8 in the wealthiest (British Heart Foundation and Stroke Association, 2009). Members of the black population of the UK (such as Eric and Barbara), have a strikingly increased incidence of stroke that is independent of their socio-economic status (Wolfe et al., 2002). South Asian people who have come to live in the UK have an even higher incidence of stroke (Gunaranthne et al., 2009).

The outcomes from stroke can be hard to predict. For some people even quite major strokes can be overcome and good functional recovery is possible. For other people it appears that only modest return to previous function is possible. Lalit Kalra and Rajiv Ratan (2006), two specialist stroke researchers from UK and USA respectively, reviewed some of the recent advances in stroke rehabilitation in an attempt to discern which features of rehabilitation may be responsible for ensuring the maximum recovery. They conclude that '… reorganization in the brain can occur with both recovery and learning but improves significantly in both with practice … Early mobilization is seen as one of the key components of acute stroke care responsible for good outcomes'. In summary the sooner active rehabilitation is carried out and the more intensive and supportive the interventions are, the more likely the person is to achieve their maximum potential recovery. However, in practice, both the intensity and variety of rehabilitative activity often fails to live up to these evidence-based ideals.

Five weeks after discharge from hospital Eric has attended a local Day Hospital on two occasions. A hospital minibus picked him up early in the morning. Although the distance to the hospital is not great the minibus picked up several other people for the Day Hospital en route and the journey time for Eric was over an hour each way. By the time Eric arrived for his therapy at the Day Hospital he was exhausted and he spent the day slumped in his wheelchair, almost asleep. On both occasions the speech therapist and physiotherapist at the Day Hospital decided that he was too tired to gain benefit from their attention and they left him dozing.

The difficulties that Eric and Dorothy experienced in trying to get therapy that is tailored to their specific needs are not atypical. Policy makers have been aware for many years of problems faced by people with stroke and the strain that is evident on those caring for them. This awareness led to the publication of the *National Stroke Strategy* in 2007, which was itself the culmination of many years of detailed consultation and preparation by expert committees (DH, 2007). However, the inspiring words found within official policy documents frequently fail to become implemented in practice. This situation seems especially true in the case of people with stroke during their rehabilitation phase. The National Stroke Strategy has not led to the development of universally high quality primary care and rehabilitation services. Three years after the publication of the *National Stroke Strategy* the National Audit Office and the Department of Health in England conducted a survey of 760 people with stroke or caring for people with stroke (DH, 2010):

Improvements in acute care are not yet matched by progress in delivering more effective post-hospital support for stroke survivors, where there are barriers to joint working between the health service, social care and other services such as benefits and employment support. Patients and carers also lack good information about the services they may need and how to access them on discharge from hospital, as well as on how to prevent further strokes. Only half of stroke survivors in our survey said they were given advice on further stroke prevention on leaving hospital, and only a quarter were given information about the benefits system … in 2008, 30% of patients were not given a follow-up appointment within six weeks of discharge from hospital … psychological support was rated the least satisfactory service in long-term care in our patient survey, with only 24% of respondents rating it as good or very good. (Department of Health, 2010: 8)

As well as official surveys of the quality of care that is available to people who have had a stroke and their carers there has been considerable investigation of this subject by researchers and specialist health care professionals. A picture often emerges from this research that describes services that are very patchy. In some instances people feel well served and supported by the services that are available for them, but often this is not the case and people feel rejected or abandoned.

Since discharge from hospital one 53 year old who had a stroke reported:

… since then nobody has bothered to ring at all, which is a bit annoying because when you first come out I think that's the time when you really need the physio. You need to keep it going you know … I practise my walking, because I still feel the more I do, the easier it will be … I'm sure they'd come round or refer me to somebody that could help but I don't think there is … (Ellis-Hill et al., 2009: 65–6)

The most usual conceptualization for people who have had a stroke and for their informal and professional carers is to think of the event of stroke and its sequelae as a 'loss' (McKevitt et al., 2004). For people who have had a stroke there is often a loss of physical function, perhaps a loss of role or status and frequently a perceived loss of independence. A loss of identity for the person experiencing a stroke is also a common but enormously significant finding (McKevitt et al., 2004). As well as providing the resources and support that would help people who have had a stroke recover physically to their maximum potential, services should aim to understand the nature of these losses for each individual patient and ease the process of adjustment and change of status. Professional support for these more complex psychological changes appears to be especially important:

... the uncertainty. Even now I'm not sure whether one should expect another stroke or whether you should accept that it's behind you and it's unlikely to happen again ... the biggest problem is not knowing what the future holds ... (Ellis-Hill et al., 2009: 68)

Professional health workers may also find that dealing with the transitional status of people they look after is problematic and perhaps beyond their competence (Wiles et al., 2002, 2004). In these quotes physiotherapists are talking about the ways they deal with the expectations of people who have recently had a stroke:

> ... [He] is still focused on really getting back to exactly how he was before as opposed to having accepted that he is going to be left with some residual prob-lems from the stroke and therefore adjusting his lifestyle accordingly ... It's hard to know what you can say to make the patient accept it. (Wiles et al., 2002: 847)

> ... I do think her expectations are quite high ... I think I've got to keep reinforcing every time she comes ... that she may never feel as good as she did and she may not achieve absolutely everything that she wants to. (Wiles et al., 2002: 844–5)

The challenge for health professionals is to find a balance between being realistic about the person's chances of returning to their previous level of functioning while still maintaining the morale and motivation of that indi-vidual and the people around them. The importance of motivation and positive outlook has been commented on by many researchers and also by people recovering from stroke: 'The day you give up trying to get better, that's as far as you get' (female person with a stroke aged 40, quoted in Dixon et al., 2007: 233).

Low mood, poor levels of motivation and 'apathy' were found to be both prevalent and persistent in people who have had a stroke (Mayo et al., 2009). These psychological conditions, which are often characterized by a lack of self-initiated actions, can directly affect recovery from stroke and hinder progress towards rehabilitation. Niall Maclean, a researcher at Kings College Department of Public Health Sciences and his colleagues, interviewed 22 people who had recently had strokes (Maclean et al., 2000). They found that people with stroke who worked alongside their profes-sional helpers and who shared and understood similar aims were less likely to be poorly motivated than those who were overprotected by family members or who lacked information about the recovery process.

A more recent study reported from Norway (Mangset et al., 2008) looked in detail at features of care such as respect and dignity and their relationship with rehabilitation. Although this was a hospital-based study the message is clear for primary care workers as well. The study found that people who were treated generally well and with due respect by the professional staff at the hospital also felt that their rehabilitation was satisfactory. Some others reported serious incidents of lack of respect and it is these people with stroke who fared worse:

> I'd say they don't listen to us. Not at all. They shut their ears as they pass by: 'I haven't got time now. I've got to do this and now I've got to do that'. (Mangset et al., 2008: 830)

> It has something to do with being ... with human dignity, which in itself is a problem since you're lying there and need help with everything, that you don't get sent around like a package ... you don't know what you're doing, where you're going. You really don't know a thing, which proves the point that you don't have any dignity at all.... (Mangset et al., 2008: 829)

Continuity and quality of primary care

Providing the necessary levels and standards of service for people who have had a stroke and for others within primary care settings is not an easy matter. Throughout the literature and in reports from people who have had a stroke and for their carers, however, continuity of care remains a dominant theme:

> ... I think the main thing is that [the known GP] has been there for me in the past ... it's nice to know that your GP's there ... that he's really interested in what's happening to you ... and caring about your health and concerned about your well-being, you know, it's nice to know that somebody's there. (Adam, 2007: 6)

Doctors working in primary care also value continuity in their clinical relationships with people living with long-term conditions. Ridd and his colleagues interviewed a wide range of general practitioners who reported that continuity improved trust, communication and concordance. (Ridd et al., 2007)

> ... I mean that's the point of being a GP is to have that [continuity] rather than being in Accident and Emergency and seeing someone different every day. (Ridd et al., 2007: 465)

> ... it's an ongoing commitment really, it's not a one-off consultation with an individual patient, but it's kind of something over a prolonged period of time or for which the doctor feels responsible for that patient, without a particular consultation. It also means being available, the patient knowing that the person they go to who will take that responsibility for it ... it's a kind of ongoing commitment really. (Adam, 2007: 6)

Continuity between an individual with a long-term condition and a single doctor, however, is not always without significant problems. What if the relationship is not mutually respectful or when it becomes a dependency or co-dependency? And what if the person with a long-term condition is stuck with a doctor that they don't feel takes them seriously?

> ... I had actually suffered from a bad leg for years, but I damn well did not mention it to [name of Dr.] anymore. He had laughed at me once, and he should not be allowed to do that again, should he? There have been a lot of such examples; that he almost laughed and started talking about the birds in the garden ... (Frederiksen et al., 2009: 5)

Some doctors seem unsuited for looking after people with long-term conditions and find it hard to be respectful. This quotation comes from a doctor who was training to become a general practitioner:

> ... There's also the element of there's some patients you just hate seeing, these heart-sink patients, I've already got one or two of them and you're just, they walk in the door and they say, 'Well doctor,' and you know for starters that they're never going to be well ... (Ridd et al., 2007: 465)

Eight months after his original stroke Eric can always be found in his wheelchair in his front room. His communication skills have deteriorated since his discharge from hospital and he has a persistently low mood. Barbara is worried that he hasn't been seen by his GP for a long while. In the morning before leaving for work she rings the GP surgery for a home visit that she feels is reluctantly accepted by the receptionist who takes her call. Later in the day a young doctor they have never seen before comes to the house. She does not introduce herself, but measures Eric's blood pressure and takes some blood from his arm.

People recovering from stroke are not, of course, entirely dependent on the relationship with their general practitioner. Both physiotherapy (Robison et al., 2009), and occupational therapy (Gilbertson et al., 2000), have been shown to be helpful in supporting people who have had a stroke in the period after they have returned home. These resources are not universally available and they are almost always time-limited. People may be offered a set number of sessions with a specialist therapist during which time progress might be apparent, but problems often occur when the sessions have to end. Rose Wiles, a sociologist from Southampton and her colleagues describe this phase as *'the management of disappointment'*, at which time the person with a stroke and their carers might feel acute distress and abandonment (Wiles et al., 2004).

Psychological and emotional support for people who have had a stroke and for their carers is often entirely lacking or found to be of insufficient quantity or quality. The Healthcare Commission surveys in 2004 and 2006 found that large numbers of people felt that they had not received enough help and support with emotional problems either in hospital or in the time following their discharge:

> ... it was not explained to me that as well as the physical damage that a stroke can cause, there are also emotional ones. I was fortunate that the physical damage was very small, but the loss of personal drive and desire to work was very hard to take. (Healthcare Commission, 2006: 16)

Managerial responses aimed to improve the quality of care for people with stroke within primary care

Professional health care workers throughout the NHS as well as managers at all levels have long been aware of the deficiencies and lack of consistency of care for people who have had a stroke both in hospital and on their return home. Poor levels of help, support and information for their family and for their informal carers have also been perceived as a major problem. But how can a centralized NHS management team improve services and ensure consistently high levels of care? One important managerial initiative within the NHS has been the production of the *National Stroke Strategy* (DH, 2007). This document is the product of many years of debate and deliberation by managers, professionals and consultation with people who use the services. It details the aspirations for a gold standard of care for people who have had a stroke and for their carers.

Within the primary care services the managerial response has been more specific and focused on the production of clinical targets that general practitioners and primary care teams should meet in order to improve their care of people who have had a stroke. These targets have been enshrined in the Quality and Outcomes Framework (QOF) which is a mechanism through which primary care teams receive payment for meeting specific targets.

The Quality and Outcomes Framework (QOF) clinical criteria for stroke and transient ischaemic attacks are set out in Table 7.1. The difficulty in trying to lay down guidelines that improve the quality of care is immediately apparent. Most of the complex issues that have been outlined in this chapter that affect the actual and perceived quality of care for people who have had a stroke are missing from the list. The list of clinical requirements within QOF has become a reductionist version of the minimum that a competent primary care team should do for the people they are looking after. A primary care team who gave support to the person and their relatives and carers, who engage at an emotional level and make sure that all possible rehabilitation services are provided, would receive no additional

Table 7.1   QOF clinical domain – stroke and transient ischaemic attacks

	Records	Points
1	The Practice can produce a register of patients with Stroke or TIA	4
2	The percentage of new patients with presumptive stroke who have been referred for confirmation of the diagnosis by CT or MRI scan	2
	Ongoing Management	
3	The percentage of patients with TIA or stroke who have a record of smoking status in the last 15 months, except those who have never smoked where smoking status should be recorded at least once since diagnosis	3
4	The percentage of patients with a history of TIA or stroke who smoke and whose notes contain a record that smoking cessation advice or referral to a specialist service, if available, has been offered in the last 15 months	2
5	The percentage of patients with TIA or stroke who have a record of blood pressure in the notes in the preceding 15 months	2
6	The percentage of patients with a history of TIA or stroke in whom the last blood pressure reading (measured in last 15 months) is 150/90 or less	5
7	The percentage of patients with TIA or stroke who have a record of total cholesterol in the last 15 months	2
8	The percentage of patients with TIA or stroke whose last measured total cholesterol (measured in last 15 months) is 5 mmol/l or less	5
9	The percentage of patients with a stroke shown to be non-haemorrhagic, or a history of TIA, who have a record that aspirin, an alternative anti-platelet therapy, or an anti-coagulant is being taken (unless a contraindication or side-effects are recorded)	4
10	The percentage of patients with TIA or stroke who have had influenza immunization in the preceding 1 September to 31 March	2
	Total Points	31

payment at all. A primary care team 'ticking all the boxes' would receive about £4,000 for completing a very basic checklist.

The introduction of payments under the Quality and Outcomes Framework has led to changes in the way that people are looked after by primary care teams throughout the UK. Kath Checkland and her colleagues studied primary care teams in England and Scotland following the introduction of the new incentives for health care. They identified a 'real shift towards the delivery of a more biomedical, disease-orientated model of care occurring in response to the imperatives embodied in the new contract' (Checkland et al., 2008: 799). Their research, however, focused on even more uncomfortable findings;

> In spite of the real changes occurring in their practices towards a more bio-medical model of care, the doctors in our study seemed unaware of this, denying that significant change had taken place … They maintained discursive claims to holistic practice, using a variety of different arguments to demonstrate how they continued to care for 'whole people'… . In spite of the ubiquity of GP claims to holism and patient-centeredness, definitions of what this means in practice have remained vague and slippery… [and] this definitional slipperiness provided space

within which clinicians could claim holism whilst engaging in working practices based on a quite different philosophy. (Checkland et al., 2008: 799)

Even within a biomedical framework the collection of data on which payments to primary care teams depend seems to be of variable quality and open to manipulation or 'gaming'. For example if a doctor or practice nurse takes someone's blood pressure and the reading is not within the clinical guidelines that would trigger incentive payments, who would be able to check whether the figure recorded in that person's notes is accurate or not? There is some evidence to show that recorded values since the new contract have become clustered below the QOF target (Carey et al., 2009) and that some people for whom targets cannot be reached are excluded from QOF reporting altogether (Gubb and Li, 2008).

The unintended consequences following introduction of new ways of paying general practitioners to improve the quality of the care they provide remain under scrutiny. In addition to the 'gaming' and manipulation of reported statistics for financial gain some of the relationships within primary care teams have changed. There has been a growth in administrative tasks within primary care to collect data and practice nurses may feel resentful that they are doing most of the work that triggers additional incentive payments, but not sharing in the financial benefits that the practice receives. One practice nurse claims:

> … I'm sure that we haven't had our salary updated as much as we should, for the money that they're probably getting from QOF… we're doing a lot more of their work for them, and not much in the way of money recognition … (Campbell et al., 2005: 230)

Integrated services for people who have had a stroke

Approximately one year after Eric's first stroke his condition deteriorated quite suddenly and he was admitted to hospital. He was found to have a urinary tract infection which was treated quickly and he was discharged after a few days. On this occasion he was referred to a stroke family care worker who was responsible for organizing and co-ordinating a range of services that both Eric and Barbara continue to enjoy.

Successful rehabilitation after a stroke and a return to as many previously valued activities as possible can be a complex task that depends on the skills and enthusiasm of professional and informal carers (Robison et al., 2009). In some geographical areas the necessary specialist services may not have been established and, even where a network of services is available, people with stroke and their informal carers may not be aware of them. Even professional workers may not know how to access the services that would help the people for whom they have responsibility.

Mant et al. (2005) asked a wide range of people who had had a stroke, as well as their carers, what they wanted and needed from community services:

> … Three major themes emerged: the prominence of psychological and emotional issues; lack of information available for stroke patients and their carers; and the central role of primary care as a point of contact with services. (Mant et al., 2005: 135)

For Eric and Barbara the psychological and emotional issues following Eric's stroke had become almost as significant as the physical problems. As soon as they realized that someone (the stroke family care worker) was interested in them as individuals and that there may be additional sources of help they felt better and were able to take a more active part in making necessary caring arrangements for themselves.

A systematic review (Smith et al., 2008) found evidence that the provision of information to people and their carers about stroke increased their satisfaction and lowered depression scores. The evidence for effectiveness for stroke liaison workers is hard to analyse (Ellis et al., 2010), because each individual person who has had a stroke has such different, and potentially complex, needs. Jonathan Mant and his colleagues (2005), found, however, that family support increased social activities and improved the quality of life for carers six months after the stroke.

Not all services for people who have had a stroke are based on formal or statutory provision. The Stroke Association provides extensive information about preventing stroke and how to cope with a stroke. The association runs more than 500 Stroke Clubs throughout the UK.

> Prompted by their support worker Eric and Barbara started to attend their local Stroke Club. A volunteer driver picks them up and they spend a few hours at the club each week. They have found that the club is a good way for them to be in touch with other people in similar circumstances. They have made new friends. Eric has found that he can do more activities than he thought he was able to previously. He's learnt how to use his left hand to play bowls.

Summary

This chapter has considered stroke as a long-term condition that affects an estimated 150,000 people each year in the UK. Although there have been improvements in the acute care of people who have had a stroke, rehabilitation efforts have lagged behind. Services for people who have had a stroke are often imperfectly delivered and are not universally available. Some centralized initiatives, such as performance payments for general practitioners, have had unintended consequences and may not have improved the quality of care for people who have had a stroke or for their carers. Campaigning and support organizations, such as the Stroke Association can do a lot to improve the lives of people with stroke.

Further reading

Stroke Association: http://www.stroke.org.uk/about_us/index.html
Department of Health (2007) *National Stroke Strategy.* London: The Stationery Office. [Online] Available at: http://www.dh.gov.uk/en/Publicationsandstatistics/Publications/PublicationsPolicyAndGuidance/DH_081062

References

Adam, R. (2007) '"Personal Care" and general practice medicine in the UK: A qualitative interview study with patients and general practitioners', *Osteopathic Medicine and Primary Care*, 1: 13.

British Heart Foundation and Stroke Association (2009) *Stroke Statistics.* London: British Heart Foundation.

Campbell, S., McDonald, R. and Lister, H. (2008) 'The experience of Pay for Performance in English Family Practice: a qualitative study', *Annals of Family Medicine*, 6 (3): 228–34.

Carey, I., Nightingale, C.M., DeWilde, S., Harris, T., Whincup, P.H. and Cook, D.G. (2009) 'Blood pressure recording bias during a period when the Quality and Outcomes Framework was introduced', *Journal of Human Hypertension*, 23(11): 764–70.

Checkland, K., Harrison, S., McDonald, R., Grant, S., Campbell, S. and Guthrie, B. (2008) 'Biomedicine, holism and general medical practice: Responses to the 2004 General Practice contract', *Sociology of Health and Illness*, 30 (5): 788–803.

Department of Health (2007) *National Stroke Strategy.* London: The Stationery Office.

Department of Health and National Audit Office (2010) *Progress in Improving Stroke Care.* London: The Stationery Office.

Dixon, G., Thornton, E. and Young, C. (2007) 'Perceptions of self-efficacy and rehabilitation among neurologically disabled adults', *Clinical Rehabilitation*, 21: 230–40.

Ellis, G., Mant, J., Langhorne, P., Dennis, M. and Winner, S. (2010) 'Stroke liaison workers for stroke patients and carers: An individual patient data meta-analysis', *Cochrane Database Systematic Review*, 12(5): CD005066.

Ellis-Hill, C., Robison, J., Wiles, R., McPherson, K., Hyndman, D. and Ashburn, A. (2009) 'Going home to get on with life: Patients and carers experiences of being discharged from hospital following a stroke', *Disability and Rehabilitation*, 31(2): 61–72.

Frederiksen, H., Kragstrup, J. and Dehlholm-Lambertsen, G. (2009) 'It's all about recognition! Qualitative study of the value of interpersonal continuity in general practice', *BMC Family Practice*, 10: 47.

Gilbertson, L., Langhorne, P., Walker, A., Allen, A. and Murray, G. (2000) 'Domiciliary occupational therapy for patients with stroke discharged from hospital: Randomised controlled trial', *British Medical Journal*, 320: 603–6.

Gubb, J. and Li, G. (2008) *Checking up on Doctors: A Review of the Quality and Outcomes Framework for General Practitioners.* London: Civitas – Institute for the Study of Civil Society.

Gunarathne, A. et al. (2009) 'Ischaemic stroke in South Asians', *Stroke,* 40:415–23.

Healthcare Commission (2006) *Survey of Patients 2006: Caring for People After They Have Had a Stroke. A Follow-up Survey of Patients.* London: Commission for Healthcare Audit and Inspection.

Kalra, L. and Ratan, R. (2006) 'Recent advances in stroke rehabilitation', *Stroke,* 38: 235–7.

Maclean, N., Pouind, P., Wolfe, C. and Rudd, A. (2000) 'Qualitative analysis of stroke patients' motivation for rehabilitation', *British Medical Journal,* 321: 1051–4.

Mangset, M., Dahl, T., Forde, R. and Wyller, T. (2008) '"We're just sick people, nothing else": … factors contributing to elderly stroke patients' satisfaction with rehabilitation', *Clinical Rehabilitation,* 22: 825–35.

Mant, J., Carter, J., Wade, D., Winner, S., Roche, J and Wade, D. (2005) 'Family support for stroke: One year follow up of a randomised controlled trial', *Journal of Neurology, Neurosurgery and Psychiatry,* 76: 1006–8.

Mayo, N., Fellows, L.K., Scott, S.C., Cameron, J. and Wood-Dauphinee, S. (2009) 'A longitudinal view of apathy and its impact after stroke', *Stroke,* 40: 3299–307.

McKevitt, C., Redfern, J., Mold, F. and Wolfe, C. (2004) 'Qualitative studies of stroke: A systematic review', *Stroke*, 35: 1499–505.

Ridd, M., Shaw, A. and Salisbury, C. (2007) '"Two sides of the coin" – the value of personal continuity to GPs: A qualitative interview study', *Family Practice*, 23: 461–8.

Robison, J., Wiles, R., Ellis-Hill, C., McPherson, K., Hyndman, D. and Ashburn, A. (2009) 'Resuming previously valued activities post-stroke: Who or what helps?' *Disability and Rehabilitation,* 31(19): 1555–66.

Smith, J., Forster, A., House, A., Knapp, P., Wright, J. and Young, J. (2008) 'Information provision for stroke patients and their caregivers', *Cochrane Database Systematic Review,* 16(2): CD001919.

Wiles, R., Ashbuirn, A., Payne, S. and Murphy, C. (2002) 'Patients' expectations of recovery following stroke: a qualitative study', *Disability and Rehabilitation,* 24(16): 841–50.

Wiles, R., Ashburn, A., Payne, S. and Murphy, C. (2004) 'Discharge from physiotherapy following stroke: The management of disappointment', *Social Science and Medicine,* 59: 1263–73.

Wolfe, C., Rudd, A.G., Howard, R., Coshall, C., Stewart, J., Lawrence, E., Hajat, C. and Hillen, T. (2002) 'Incidence and case fatality rates of stroke subtypes in a multi-ethnic population: The South London Stroke Register', *Journal of Neurology, Neurosurgery and Psychiatry,* 72: 211–16.

8

Diabetes and Pregnancy: Service-users' Perspectives on Services and on Research

Cathy E. Lloyd and Sarah Earle

> **Overview**
>
> - Diabetes in pregnancy – what are the risks?
> - Medical care for women with diabetes during pregnancy
> - The importance of psychosocial factors
> - Service users' perspectives: Qualitative accounts
> - Service users' experiences and involvement in the research process
> - Future research and practice: Ways forward

Diabetes is the most common medical complication in pregnancy and is associated with an increased risk of obstetric complications, including congenital abnormalities, increased rates of caesarean delivery and perinatal mortality (CEMACH, 2007). Diabetes is a long-term condition for which there is no cure but there are recommendations for ways it can be managed (Department of Health, 2001). Type 1 diabetes occurs in childhood or early adulthood and necessitates the use of multiple daily insulin injections and testing of blood sugar levels in order to maintain health and well-being. Type 2 diabetes typically occurs later in life, is associated with being overweight, and is treated with diet and increased physical activity initially.

Medication and/or insulin injections are often required. Gestational diabetes (GDM) – diabetes which occurs during pregnancy – happens when the body cannot produce enough insulin to meet the extra needs of pregnancy. It is associated with being overweight and also with a family history of Type 2 diabetes. Although it usually goes away after childbirth, women with GDM have an increased risk of developing Type 2 diabetes later on in life as well as having GDM in subsequent pregnancies. Both Type 2 diabetes and GDM are more common in women from minority ethnic groups. Having diabetes means having to incorporate a whole range of self-care behaviours into daily life: blood testing, medication taking and dietary restrictions, to name but a few. People with diabetes are at greater risk of developing heart disease, eye and kidney disease, and are also more likely to have mental health problems – such as depression – compared with people without this condition.

During pregnancy and childbirth, diabetes (whatever its type) introduces a range of challenges for both the women themselves and those providing their care. Current recommendations for the care of women with diabetes before and during pregnancy focus on medical considerations, especially achieving tight blood glucose control. The main aim of this care is to reduce the risk of complications during pregnancy and childbirth. However, the psychosocial impact of pre-natal care for women with diabetes in pregnancy is less well recognized and has only recently begun to be considered. This chapter provides an overview of current practice with regard to the care of women with diabetes during pregnancy and childbirth. Using the available empirical evidence, the experiences of the mothers and their families are considered and ways forward for future research and practice are recommended.

Diabetes in pregnancy: What are the risks?

Rates of diabetes during pregnancy are rapidly increasing and are seen to be a serious public health concern (CEMACH, 2007). These increased rates are mainly due to the rapid rise in the number of women who have Type 2 diabetes and it has been suggested that this is associated with an increased prevalence of overweight and obesity (Coulthard et al., 2008). Outcomes for women with diabetes during pregnancy tend to be measured in terms of biomedical markers of morbidity such as congenital abnormalities, and mortality. A key report from the Confidential Enquiry into Maternal and Child Health which focused on women with pre-existing diabetes, highlighted a five-fold increase in still-births, a three-fold increased risk of perinatal mortality and a two-fold increased risk of congenital abnormalities (CEMACH, 2010). Preterm delivery rates were more than five times more common in women with diabetes compared to women without this condition, and caesarian section rates were nearly trebled. Research suggests that women who develop gestational diabetes also have an increased risk of morbidity and mortality. Barahona and colleagues (2005), for example, note that gestational diabetes was a predictor for adverse maternal outcomes including hypertension, and adverse neonatal outcomes including prematurity, low Apgar scores and perinatal mortality. However, adverse outcomes are more significant for women with pre-existing diabetes compared to women who develop diabetes in pregnancy. The concerns noted in the CEMACH report are reflected in the current National Institute for Health and Clinical Excellence (NICE) recommendation that screening for gestational diabetes should be offered to women with certain identified risk factors, including a body mass index over 30 and any first degree relative with diabetes (NICE, 2008).

Medical care for women with diabetes during pregnancy

The CEMACH enquiry reported the results of their investigations into the standards of medical care provided to women with diabetes during pregnancy in Wales, Northern Ireland and England. Both pre-conception care and clinical care during pregnancy were found to be lacking; in particular issues of 'suboptimal' fetal surveillance and poor management of maternal risks were identified and found to be associated with poor outcomes. This report underlines the strong focus on biomedical markers of pregnancy outcome that remains at the forefront of services, with little if any consideration of wider psychosocial concerns.

Whilst clinical outcomes for both mother and child remain poorer for women with diabetes compared to those without diabetes, there are some signs that diabetes management during pregnancy is improving (Waddingham, 2008). Two years ago the National Institute for Health and Clinical Excellence (NICE) issued guidance for the care of women with diabetes during pregnancy which spell out in detail the physiological and biomedical management of diabetes before, during and after pregnancy. There is significant evidence to suggest that such management reduces both neonatal and maternal morbidity and mortality (for example, see Crowther et al., 2005; Gabb and Graves, 2003). These guidelines have paved the way to more standardized care by providing a template for care protocols throughout the UK. Recent research suggests that although diabetes management in pregnancy might be improving, this improvement is not uniform across the UK (Williams and Modder, 2010).

Although remaining almost exclusively focused on biomedical care, the NICE guidance does acknowledge, early on in the report, the need to 'take into account women's needs and preferences'. The report argues that 'Women with diabetes should have the opportunity to make their informed decisions about their care and treatment, in partnership with their healthcare professionals' (NICE, 2008: 6). Although we take the viewpoint here that the psychosocial needs of women with diabetes during pregnancy are more often than not overlooked, this is not to say that, in our experience, women want their biomedical and physiological needs ignored or even placed as secondary. Indeed women have considerably high expectations of maternity care services in relation to its ability to reduce, or eradicate, foetal abnormalities or neonatal mortality and morbidity (Hildingsson et al., 2002), especially following prior experiences of pregnancy loss (Robson et al., 2009). Rather, as will be discussed below, many women report their concern to *integrate* the two aspects so that a more holistic approach to care is promoted.

The importance of psychosocial factors

As noted above, diabetes imposes a range of care needs on the person with the condition. In pregnant women this means having to incorporate self-management behaviours such as frequent blood testing and medication taking into their daily lives, which have hitherto not been part of their experience. At the same time, they can expect to be closely monitored by a range of health care professionals throughout their pregnancy. Biomedical concern for the well-being of both mother and baby is not without its challenges however and women's psychosocial well-being may be compromised.

The *National Service Framework for Diabetes* highlighted the importance of optimizing the outcomes of pregnancy through empowering and supporting women with diabetes:

> Standard 9: The NHS will develop, implement and monitor policies that seek to empower and support women with pre-existing diabetes and those who develop diabetes during pregnancy to optimize the outcomes of their pregnancy. (Department of Health, 2001)

Although this policy recommendation has been one of the cornerstones of diabetes care for nearly a decade, little remains known about the psychosocial experiences of women with diabetes during pregnancy. Recently it has been acknowledged that ways of improving the quality of care for women with diabetes in pregnancy still needs attention (NICE, 2008). However challenges remain in terms of putting these recommendations into practice and achieving successful clinical outcomes in pregnancy alongside psychosocial ones (Holt, 2008).

Different settings for care may influence women's perceptions of their care and whether or not a positive experience of health care services is reported. The picture is further complicated by the necessity to address the particular needs of the local community served by both primary and secondary care. Gestational diabetes is more common in women from minority ethnic groups (Deparment of Health, 2001), and there may be differences in the experiences of pregnancy according to ethnicity (Kim et al., 2007). However this remains unclear as most UK studies do not include non-English speaking individuals and so their views remain unknown. Of the research that does exist, the picture that emerges is complex. For example, Katbamna (2000), who focused on the distinctive cultural practices of Gujurati and Bangladeshi women having babies in the UK, argued that services did not always recognize women's distinct cultural preferences. In contrast, in a review of statistical data on childbirth and ethnicity, Parsons et al. (1993) noted that differences between groups of women may be attributable to stereotyping and the exclusion of minority ethnic women from services, rather than from any distinct cultural differences between women. The work of Bowes and Domokos (2003) – who conducted a comparative study of the childbirth experiences of Pakistani women and white working class women in the UK – supports both viewpoints, concluding that there were commonalities *and* distinctions in women's experiences attributable to differences such as ethnicity and class. Other research has indicated that there are cultural differences in experience, with South Asian women being more influenced by family and religion compared to their white Caucasian counterparts (Murphy et al., 2010). A recent report has also highlighted the low take-up of health services among minority ethnic groups and stressed the need for more diverse provision (Stuart, 2008). Alongside this, consultation with minority ethnic groups and involvement in the design of services remains low (Begum, 2006).

In order to improve services for women during pregnancy we would argue that more evidence is required; evidence that should come from services users from a range of backgrounds and experiences. Indeed other research suggests that service users, when asked, can offer very creative – and cost effective – ideas for service improvement. A qualitative study exploring culturally sensitive continence care among South Asian Indian women, for example, found that women's suggestions for service improvement were relatively modest in terms of additional resource requirements (Doshani et al., 2007). Furthermore a range of data collection methods should be used in order to obtain as broad a picture as possible. Investigation of the health care experiences of women with diabetes during pregnancy can provide vital opportunities to improve both medical and psychosocial outcomes, and can inform health service provision. We have found that women who have diabetes during their pregnancies are very willing to have their voices heard and to divulge their experiences. This is in line with moves to encourage greater user-involvement in the research process itself and supports the idea that many women are keen to be involved in the design and conducting of research in this field.

To this end, we invited women with diabetes who had recently had a baby to meet with us on an informal basis to discuss their experiences as well as help us to identify what the key aspects of future research should be and how best they thought their voices could be heard. We outline some of those discussions below.

Researching service users' experiences: Qualitative reports

Clear care pathways for the clinical management of diabetes during pregnancy have been developed by specialists in pregnancy and diabetes at the NHS Trust where we met women who had had GDM, or Type 1 or Type 2 diabetes during their pregnancy. However, little was (and remains) known about the psychosocial experiences of these women, in particular with regard to their perceptions of a successful outcome of pregnancy complicated by diabetes. It was our aim to hear about those experiences, as well as to discuss with women what the priorities for research should be. The ensuing discussions were used in the design and preparation of a research proposal to investigate the experiences of women with diabetes during pregnancy and childbirth.

Our discussions with women with diabetes during pregnancy demonstrated that there were high expectations of service provision; however this was reported as often unfulfilled in practice. Problematic relationships with health care professionals were highlighted; especially the lack of rapport between patient and professional over an extended period of time. This was identified as particularly difficult during pregnancy because the women were expected to attend ante-natal clinic approximately every two weeks. It was clear that each woman responded to and developed relationships with the different health care professionals working in the diabetes ante-natal clinic in specific ways, with some women preferring a female doctor, and others preferring what was described as a 'medical approach' where the focus was mainly on blood sugar levels. Other women were clear that they wanted more from their ante-natal care than what they perceived as an over-riding concern with the medical management of diabetes:

> '... the diabetes side was fantastic, but may be just a bit more support with just being pregnant.'

> 'It [the diabetes] just dominates the pregnancy all the way through, takes all the joy out of it.'

> 'Immediately you become high risk – it's in your notes. You'll probably be ... induced early and it just changes everything so quickly.'

All the women we spoke to, regardless of their type of diabetes, reported feeling that the health care professionals' over-riding concern was with their diabetes, in particular blood glucose levels and insulin treatment, at the expense of a more positive experience of pregnancy and childbirth. Some women attended diabetes ante-natal clinics that were jointly run between the diabetologist and the obstetrician, and these were perceived to be a positive development in service delivery, particularly because of improved communication between the two health care professionals. Some of these issues were highlighted by Lawson and Rajaram (1994) over 15 years ago who noted that women struggled with the various possible definitions of their pregnancy as 'normal', 'abnormal' or 'illness'.

Many of the women reported only seeing health care professionals in the secondary care setting, and did not have access to a community midwife during pregnancy. Not only did this reinforce the medicalized nature of their pregnancy, it also engendered feelings of isolation as they spent their time in large busy hospital clinics, rather than at more local primary care settings. This, of course, further reinforces the feeling of being 'different' to other pregnant women, as noted by Thomas (2003) in her study of pregnancy and chronic illness. The majority of the participants were in favour of the development of an alternative support system for mothers-to-be, describing this as a 'buddying' system. This would involve linking mothers who had experienced diabetes during pregnancy with new or expectant mothers. One woman had experienced something similar, albeit *ad hoc*:

> 'They gave my name to a young girl and she phoned me at home – I can't remember her name – she was a godsend as I hadn't a clue what was going on. We were going through the same things, we were the same kind of age and that really helped.'

Not all the women felt they would use such a system, particularly because they felt the need to rely more on professional health care and advice when it came to managing their diabetes. More education from health care professionals on aspects such as diet was also identified as important by women. These issues raise the notion of difference between the role of authoritative and experiential knowledge in pregnancy and childbirth, and highlights the need for more social support during pregnancy for some women.

Experiences of labour were varied but overwhelmingly the clinical need (of health professionals) to maintain close monitoring of blood sugar levels was seen as problematic and impinging on all aspects of care. The difference between ante-natal care, where the responsibility for blood sugar control lay with the mothers, and care during labour, where control was taken away from mothers (and involved intravenous infusion, sliding scales of insulin, and so on) was stark. For example:

'I had one (a drip) in each hand, disabling really.'

'I had two drips in … they made me walk all down the ward into the lift with these drips on trolleys…'

Knowledge about the need for dietary intake to be balanced with insulin levels, both during and after pregnancy, and the impact on breastfeeding were both areas identified as requiring further improvement within secondary care. A number of the women were separated from their baby immediately after the birth, or very shortly after, when they were sent to the special care baby unit for further monitoring. For example:

'they didn't take her off straight away – so we did have her for about an hour … that was hard there were three women with their babies crying all night (in the ward room she shared) then there's me. I felt like I didn't have a baby.'

As noted earlier, whilst the joint diabetes/obstetric service during pregnancy was seen as a positive aspect of service development, the same could not be said in relation to women's experiences of labour and post-natal care. Here, a gap between information received from diabetologists and information from midwives and obstetricians was still in evidence, highlighting the differences between different teams and professions, as well as between generalists and specialists, as the following quotes highlight:

'When you're in labour … it would have been nice to have a diabetes nurse or doctor to reassure you that everything's alright … although I had the drip in I don't remember anyone talking to me about my diabetes.'

'My insulin drip came out and no one seemed sure whether they should put I back in or not.'

'On the labour ward when my blood sugar was so high, nobody there knew why it was and what to do about it … you've got a new baby who needs attention but your blood sugars are through the roof…'

What is interesting here is that a contrasting picture emerges from that experienced during pregnancy. During pregnancy, the 'diabetic condition' is placed centre stage in the management of women with diabetes, but during labour, diabetes is relegated and the condition of pregnancy comes to the fore. It suggests that women may wish neither the pregnancy nor the diabetes to dominate, but that they desire a holistic, integrated approach where both 'conditions' co-exist.

Service users' experiences and involvement in the research process

We held three meetings for women to attend and give us their views, and most attended with their babies (ranging in age from 6 weeks to 6 months old), which ensured a high degree of informality and encouraged a spirit of camaraderie between women. Many of the women had voiced their relief that they were able to bring their baby, as being unable to do so would have excluded them from participating. Indeed it could be argued that much research that is conducted takes place in settings where it is seen as inappropriate to bring children or babies. The women also agreed that joining in the discussions could be of benefit both to them and to other women with diabetes:

'I think it's good to share views and to give feedback really on our experiences through pregnancy, and if we can help other mums who are pregnant at the moment or will be, I think it benefits them.'

None of the women we met had been involved in health services research in the past, but all were interested in being involved in a range of ways in the development of a research proposal to investigate issues around diabetes and pregnancy. A range of suggestions for research topics were identified, including investigating the use of induction at 38 weeks, researching the experiences of women with different types of diabetes, and identifying ways of sharing stories of diabetes during pregnancy.

All the women made suggestions in terms of protocol design, and half were interested in being involved in other aspects of the research process including data collection and belonging to an 'investigative team'. Alternative ways of collecting data were discussed with both quantitative and qualitative methods considered. The women identified surveys as a useful method of collecting data, particularly if people wished to remain anonymous. Discussion or focus groups were seen as a useful way to share experiences. All those contacted after these discussions reported feeling pleased that they continued to be consulted and that their feedback was important in developing future ideas for research.

A first draft of a grant proposal to research women's experiences of diabetes and pregnancy was circulated to all the women who had indicated they would like to comment on it. Both the content and the layout of the proposal were commented on.

'I've reviewed and feel that the content is good, it explains what the research is aiming to do and it has a lot of meaningful information. I feel that the layout could be improved and have made comments below.'

'Would it be appropriate to put somewhere in the value for money section about the potential to assist with diet control (by improved support) and hence reduced costs to NHS throughout pregnancy and birth – seems to me that insulin controlled = early induction = increased likelihood of c-section = ditto for future pregnancies.'

'I think this is an excellent project and I do hope you get funding as it could make a huge difference to the care given to expectant ladies who unfortunately develop GDM ...'

Although the women we approached were keen to be involved in research in a range of ways as described above, less than half (13/30) of those initially approached were actually able to meet with us face-to-face. For those we were able to contact, poor turnout on the day was mostly due to illness which is to be expected in this group (i.e. women with young babies). All those who attended were English-speaking, so the views of those who were non-English speaking were not obtained. Future research clearly needs to ensure that the voices of service users from minority ethnic groups are heard. Our previous research in the area of diabetes has demonstrated that it is possible to engage with individuals from South Asian communities, particularly if qualitative methods of research, such as focus groups, are used (Lloyd et al., 2008).

A review of service user involvement in health care notes that the benefits for participants is often on a personal level, including gaining knowledge and experience, an improved sense of well-being, self-esteem and confidence (Minogue et al., 2005). However, as the same review points out, working collaboratively with service users is not always straightforward, and there is a tendency to omit service users from planning and priority-setting. Thompson et al. (2009) note that some health services researchers are quite anxious about involving service users, and the public more generally, in research and that whilst this is encouraged by the Department of Health (and other potential funders) the number of health researchers actually involving the public in research is fairly limited.

Future research and practice: Ways forward

There are clear guidelines for the clinical care of women with diabetes during pregnancy and childbirth. However the wider psychosocial experience of pregnancy remains less researched. Our work has demonstrated the possibilities of working with service users in order to begin to develop better quality services in secondary care. Reconciling the concerns of service users with those of health care professionals, of course, can be challenging and this has been highlighted here. For example, some women wanted health care professionals to focus more holistically on their experiences of pregnancy and childbirth rather than solely on the medical management of diabetes and the measurement of blood glucose levels.

Our research has suggested that there are benefits to a collaborative way of working, not just between health care practitioners and service users, but also with researchers. The discussions have resulted in greater understanding of women's key concerns as well as providing women with a positive opportunity to share their stories of pregnancy and childbirth and their experiences of health care. By encouraging women to voice their concerns in a non-threatening environment (which included a diabetes specialist midwife) the more traditional notion of health care professional as the person with the knowledge (and therefore power) and the service user as the passive recipient of care continues to be called into question. Challenges remain, however, in securing the engagement of service users, not just in terms of participating in health services research, but also in realizing active partnership with health care professionals.

The NSF for child and maternal health includes the recommendation that all women should have access to high quality maternity services that meet their needs (Department of Health, 2004). This includes access to information about available services in order to be able to make the most appropriate choices for care both during and after pregnancy. There remains, however, tensions between concerns with the vital medical management of diabetes and the desire for a more positive experience of pregnancy and diabetes. Previous work has highlighted communication difficulties between both health care professionals and service users as well as between different groups of professionals (CEMACH, 2007). Our work has also shown that it is possible to involve service users, such as women who have experienced diabetes during pregnancy, in health services research, and to play a key role in the development of services at the local level.

Summary

Diabetes during pregnancy is the most common medical complication in pregnancy and requires constant vigilance to monitor the biomedical outcomes. These may be at odds with the psychosocial well-being of women who have concerns other than biomedical ones in terms of how *they* define a positive and successful pregnancy experience. The voices of service users have rarely been heard, both in terms of women's experiences of pregnancy and diabetes as well as with regard to their involvement in research. This chapter reports some of the findings from a consultation process between women with diabetes during pregnancy, health care professionals and academic researchers. Although challenges remain, it is possible for women who have experienced diabetes during pregnancy to be involved in health services research, and to play a key role in the development of services at the local level.

Further reading

CEMACH (2010) *Perinatal Mortality 2008*. London: Confidential Enquiry into Maternal and Child Health (CEMACH).

Department of Health (2010) *Diabetes NSF: Six Years On. Delivering the Diabetes National Service Framework*. London: Department of Health.

Diabetes UK website available at http://www.diabetes.org.uk/

References

Barahona, M.J., Sucunza, N., Garcia-Patterson, A., Hernandez, M., Adelantado, J.M., Ginovart, G., De Leiva, A. and Corcoy, R. (2005) 'Period of gestational diabetes mellitus diagnosis and maternal and fetal morbidity', *Acta Obstetrica et Gynecologica Scandinavica*, 84(7): 622–7.

Begum, N. (2006) *Doing it for Themselves: Participation and Black and Minority Ethnic Services Users*. London: Social Care Institute for Excellence/Race Equality Unit.

Bowes, A. and Domokos, T. (2003) '"Your dignity is hung up at the door": Pakistani and white women's experiences of childbirth', in S. Earle and G. Letherby (eds), *Gender, Identity and Reproductive: Social perspectives*. Houndsmills: Palgrave.

CEMACH (2007) 'Confidential Enquiry into Maternal and Child Health', *Diabetes in Pregnancy: Are we Providing the Best Care?* London: CEMACH.

CEMACH (2010) 'Confidential Enquiry into Maternal and Child Health', *Perinatal Mortality 2008.* London: CEMACH.

Coulthard. T., Hawthorne, G., on behalf of the Northern Diabetes Pregnancy Service (2008) 'Type 2 diabetes in pregnancy; more to come?', *Practical Diabetes International,* 25(9): 359–61.

Crowther, C.A., Hiller, J.E., Moss, J.R., McPhee, A.J., Jeffries, W.S. and Robinson, J.S. (2005) 'Effect of treatment of gestational diabetes mellitus on pregnancy outcomes', *New England Journal of Medicine,* 352(24): 2477–86.

Department of Health (2001) *National Service Framework for Diabetes.* London: Department of Health.

Department of Health (2004) *Core Standards – National Service Fraemwork for Children, Young People and Maternity Services.* London: DH Publications.

Doshani, A., Pitchforth, E., Mayne, C.J. and Tincello, D.G. (2007) 'Culturally sensitive continence care: A qualitative study among South Asian Indian women in Leicester', *Family Practice,* 24(6): 585–93.

Gabbe, S.G. and Graves, C.R. (2003) 'Management of diabetes mellitus complicating pregnancy', *Obstetrics and Gynaecology,* 102(4): 857–68.

Hildingsson, I., Waldenstrom, U. and Radestad, I. (2002) 'Women's expectations on antenatal care as assessed in early pregnancy: Number of visits, continuity of caregiver and general content', *Acta Obstetrica et Gynecologica Scandinavica,* 81(2): 118–25.

Holt, R. (2008) 'Improving pregnancy outcomes for women with diabetes', *Practical Diabetes International,* 25: 172–4.

Katbamna, S. (2000) *'Race' and Childbirth.* Buckingham: Open University Press.

Kim, C., McEwen, L.N., Piette, J.D., Goewey, J., Ferrara, A. and Walker, E.A. (2007) 'Risk Perception for diabetes among women with histories of gestational diabetes mellitus', *Diabetes Care* 30: 2281–2286.

Lawson, E.J. and Rajaram, S. (1994) 'A transformed pregnancy: The psychosocial consequences of gestational diabetes', *Sociology of Health and Illness,* 16(4): 536–62.

Lloyd, C.E., Johnson, M.R.D., Mughal, S., Sturt, J.A., Collins, G.S., Roy, T., Bibi, R. and Barnett, A.H. (2008) 'Securing recruitment and obtaining informed consent in minority ethnic groups in the UK', *BMC Health Services Research,* 8: 68.

Minogue, V., Boness, J., Brown, A. and Girdlestone, J. (2005) 'The impact of service user involvement in research', *International Journal of Health Care Quality Assurance,* 18(2): 103–12.

Murphy, H.R., Temple, R.C., Ball, V.E., Roland, J.M., Steel, S., Zill-E-Huma, R., Simmons, D., Royce, L.R. and Skinner, T.C. (2010) 'Personal experiences of women with diabetes who do not attend pre-pregnancy care', *Diabetic Med,* 27: 92–100.

NICE (2008) *Diabetes in Pregnancy: Management of Diabetes and its Complications from Pre-conception to the Post-natal Period.* Clinical Guideline 63. [Online] Available at: www.nice.org.uk. London: National Institute of Health and Clinical Excellence

Parsons, L., MacFarlane, A. and Golding, J. (1993) 'Pregnancy, birth and maternity care', in W.I.U. Ahmad (ed.), *'Race' and Health in Contemporary Britain.* Buckingham: Open University Press.

Robson, S.J., Leader, L.R., Dear, K.B.G. and Bennett, M.J. (2009) 'Women's expectations of management in their next pregnancy after an unexplained stillbirth: An

Internet-based empirical study', *Australian and New Zealand Journal of Obstetrics and Gynaecology*, 49: 642–6.

Stuart, O. (2008) *User Participation in Health-care Services*. A Race Equality Foundation Briefing Paper. London: Race Equality Foundation.

Thomas, H. (2003) 'Pregnancy, illness and the concept of career', *Sociology of Health & Illness*, 25(5): 383–407.

Thompson, J., Barber, R., Ward, P.R., Boote, J.D., Cooper, C.L., Argmitage, C.J. and Jones, G. (2009) 'Health researchers' attitudes towards public involvement in health research', *Health Expectations*, 12(2): 209–20.

Waddingham, S. (2008) 'Looking after women with diabetes during pregnancy', *The British Journal of Primary Care Nursing*, 5. [Online] Available at: http://www.bjpcn-cardiovascular.com/download/3086

Williams, A. and Modder, J. (2010) 'Management of pregnancy complicated by diabetes: Maternal glycaemic control during pregnancy and neonatal management', *Early Human Development*, 86(5): 269–73.

9

Coeliac Disease: Psychosocial Factors in Adults and Children

Ruth A. Howard, G. Urquhart Law and Jane L. Petty

Overview

- The psychosocial consequences of living with and managing coeliac disease
- Dietary self-management and psychological well-being in children, young people and adults with the condition: Current research
- Recommendations for further research and interventions

Coeliac disease diagnosis and its management

Coeliac disease is an autoimmune condition triggered by gluten, a protein found in many foods. All of us carry a naturally occurring enzyme called tissue transglutaminase (tTG). People with coeliac disease develop anti-tTG antibodies which react to the presence of gluten in the diet and trigger the immune system. T-cells in the immune system then mistakenly attack the small intestine, causing inflammation and damage. The intestine is lined with small, finger-like projections called villi which become flattened when this immune attack occurs. This damage, known as *villous atrophy*, restricts the individual's ability to absorb nutrients and can lead to

Table 9.1 Symptoms of coeliac disease

'Classic' gastrointestinal symptoms	'Atypical' non-GI symptoms
Abdominal pain and distension	Fatigue and weakness
Bloating	Vitamin/mineral deficiencies (especially anaemia)
Constipation	Headaches/migraine
Diarrhoea	Joint pain
Nausea	Irritability and low mood
Vomiting	Clumsiness (ataxia)
Weight loss or weight gain	Abnormal menstrual cycle
Wind and flatulence	Mouth ulcers
	Lactose intolerance
	Low blood sugar (hypoglycaemia)

many different symptoms including abdominal pain, weight loss, constipation and fatigue.

There are four different phenotypes of coeliac disease that have been described (Rostrom et al., 2006).

1 'Classic' coeliac disease presents with gastrointestinal symptoms such as diarrhoea or abdominal bloating, and failure to thrive in children.
2 'Atypical' coeliac disease is the most prevalent form, presenting with few or no gastrointestinal symptoms but other issues such as anaemia, osteoporosis and fertility problems.
3 Individuals with 'silent' coeliac disease are completely asymptomatic but if a biopsy is taken it will show villous atrophy.
4 'Latent' coeliac disease represents individuals either with a diagnosis of coeliac disease but with a normal mucosal biopsy due to treatment with a gluten-free diet, or those individuals who currently have no damage to their intestine but will go on to develop coeliac disease in the future.

Coeliac disease may be diagnosed through a blood test; tests for one or both of the relevant antibodies (tTG and IgA) show 90–95% specificity and sensitivity for the condition. The 'gold standard' diagnostic test however is a biopsy of the duodenum, the upper part of the small intestine, to confirm the presence of damage to the villi (NICE, 2009). There is currently no cure for the condition and managing the symptoms of the disease involves removing all gluten from the diet (BSPGHAN, 2006; Ciclitira et al., 2010). Gluten is a generic term used to describe proteins found in wheat, barley and rye. The gluten-free diet involves removing foods such as bread, pasta, pastries, cakes and biscuits as well as a great number of processed foods. The availability of specialist gluten-free products both in supermarkets and on prescription has increased over the last ten years but there still remains an enormous disparity between the price of these products and the gluten-containing alternatives.

Coeliac disease is thought to affect around 1% of Western European populations, though this is increasing as the consumption of foods containing gluten increases across the world. Many of these will be undiagnosed cases due to the difficulty of recognizing the varied symptoms (see Table 9.1) and the overlap with other conditions such as irritable bowel syndrome (IBS) (Hopper et al., 2007). These difficulties mean that people often wait years for a correct diagnosis, with delays of over ten years between the onset of symptoms and correct diagnosis being typical (Gray and Papanicolas, 2010).

In addition to the distress caused by this delay in diagnosis, with patients often seeing multiple specialists over many years, there is evidence that sustained contact with gluten in people with undiagnosed or untreated coeliac disease is associated with an increased risk of serious health problems such as osteoporosis, non–Hodgkin's lymphoma and reproductive problems (NICE, 2009).

Like other autoimmune conditions, coeliac disease is more prevalent in women, with a ratio of around 2–3 female diagnoses per 1 male (Mearin, 2007). It can be diagnosed at any age, although there appears to be a peak in diagnosis rate between the ages of 40 and 60 (Feighery, 1999). The risk of developing coeliac disease is around 1 in 100 for an adult in the UK. This increases significantly to 1 in 10 if a first degree relative has the condition. This suggests that coeliac disease has a strong genetic component and a great deal of work has been carried out to try and identify the relevant genes. There is also considerable genetic overlap and increased risk of coeliac disease in people with other conditions such as diabetes, rheumatoid arthritis, and thyroid problems. Coeliac disease is also closely related to the skin condition Dermatitis Herpetiformis, which is also managed with a gluten-free diet.

Recent work by Jones and colleagues (2009) reported that gastrointestinal disorders, whilst accounting for around 10% of the clinical work of the NHS, are not always well managed and that there are very few criteria available to guide an improvement. Their recent research findings highlighted several key issues in the quality of care of coeliac disease in primary care which included prompt diagnosis, provision of timely and accurate information to patients and an emphasis on quality of life and depression. The remainder of this chapter will review the psychological and social impact of coeliac disease in both adults and children.

Children and young people with coeliac disease

Affecting around 1–3% of children and young people, coeliac disease is the most common form of food-related hypersensitivity of childhood. Given the recommended management of the condition, what challenges does the disease and its management pose for children, young people and families and what do we know about the impact of coeliac disease and the GFD on quality of life and psychosocial well-being?

Management of the Gluten-Free Diet

Coeliac disease presents a number of challenges to children, young people and families, including the identification of and help-seeking for initial symptoms, negotiation of a diagnosis and attendance at hospital appointments. However, the treatment for the condition – the GFD – is perhaps the most demanding. There are large differences in the findings of research studies that have tried to capture the extent of dietary self-management in children and young people, which are due to methodological variations, including definitions of self-management (otherwise termed 'compliance' or 'adherence'), the nature of measurements used (e.g. self-report, proxy-report or biological markers) and sampling. Published studies that have quantified dietary self-management in children and young people show that between 50–95% eat a strict GFD, while others either occasionally or almost always eat gluten-containing foods (e.g. Hopman et al., 2006). To understand why some children and young people manage their GFD well while others do not, research with a focus on adaptational processes and developmental coping has begun to identify the risk and protective factors associated with appropriate dietary self-management.

In general, young women with coeliac disease and younger children (age 10–13) are known to better manage their GFD, as are young people who received a diagnosis in childhood (compared to those identified via screening who are older and asymptomatic). The presence of typical, unpleasant symptoms at diagnosis (Fabiani et al., 2000) and disease-related knowledge in young people are also predictors of good dietary self-management. Conversely, poorer dietary management has been associated with poor knowledge of coeliac disease, being male, the adolescent years, being less likely to know others with the condition, skipping attendance at checkups, reporting unhappiness with professionals involved in one's health care, and having fewer and less severe symptoms. Recommendations made by children and young people to help improve dietary self-management include better food labelling, better availability of gluten-free foods (e.g. in supermarkets), better gluten-free choices on menus and in school canteens and better dietary advice (e.g. Roma et al., 2010). These are interesting and important findings. However, when we start to consider the daily experiences of children and adolescents living with coeliac disease and its essentially invisible nature (i.e. no external signs or markers), the developmental social interactions and challenges of childhood appear and give us a clue as to what extra practical, social and emotional burdens need to be negotiated when considering the GFD.

Olsson et al. (2008) in their Swedish study of 47 adolescents with coeliac disease used a qualitative approach to explore everyday life in relation to the GFD. Focus group results revealed a variety of social contexts in which the condition and the GFD could be dealt with and managed well and, alternatively, where coeliac disease and the GFD were more difficult to manage. The 'socially convenient' settings included home, where young people found it easier to stick to their GFD which was deemed integral to family functioning (e.g., gluten-free food readily available, family members knew about the condition). Situations outside of the home were more problematic and arose from limited social support, lack of disease-related knowledge in others, dissatisfaction with the availability and palatability of gluten-free food, and the attitudes and behaviours of others. Eating out, travelling and visiting friends created embarrassment – situations where the invisibility of coeliac disease was threatened and the GFD distinguished young people as being different from their peers. The decision to stick to the GFD or not was found to be complex and largely dependent on the nature and type of 'socially situated dilemmas' and stigma experiences of young people (Olsson et al., 2009).

Three European studies (Anson et al., 1990; Jackson et al., 1985; Roma et al., 2010) have explored the knowledge, attitudes and behaviours of parents of children with coeliac disease. Parents of children who are better at maintaining their GFD are reported to be more highly educated, belong to a higher social class, regard themselves as being more fully informed of the GFD, are less worried about general health, share dietary responsibility with their children (e.g., baking gluten-free food, making special trips to stock-up on foods not available locally), and demonstrate fewer difficulties in being able to chose gluten-free items from a menu. Across all parents – whether their children maintain a GFD or not – the majority report the diet to be a burden, a strain on the family budget, and linked to the avoidance of restaurants and travelling. Overall, greater levels of specific knowledge and understanding of coeliac disease, high levels of parental concern with regard to the disease and its potential future adverse impact, and the practical ability to manage a menu, are all positively associated with better dietary self-management.

Research findings on children and young people's management of the GFD, although somewhat limited by small sample sizes and cross-sectional designs, demonstrate the complex interplay that exists between biological, psychological and social processes. Understanding dietary self-management requires an appreciation of the intrapersonal and interpersonal dimensions of the task. For children and young people with coeliac disease, the GFD is necessary in order to protect against long-term health problems, yet, for a significant proportion, their health is at risk due to poor dietary self-management. A combination of illness and treatment beliefs, varying confidence to stick to the diet across settings (child and parent self-efficacy) and social-support variables appear central to an understanding of dietary self-management in coeliac disease. Fortunately, there exists a range of useful conceptual frameworks and models of health behaviour (e.g., social-cognitive theory, Bandura, 1997; self-regulation model, Leventhal et al., 2005) that can guide researchers and clinicians in the identification, assessment and manipulation of key variables, to further explore, understand and enhance self-care, including dietary self-management. The integration of such models has the potential to provide a more complete explanation of health behaviours (Hagger, 2010), and this is already advancing our understanding of dietary management in other paediatric long-term conditions (e.g. Nouwen et al., 2009).

Numerous studies have now identified the antecedents of adult health and illness behaviour as lying in childhood, and there is recognition of the interrelatedness of development and coping (Schmidt et al., 2003). If managing the GFD is an aspect of coping, then future research needs to examine how aspects of development influence it and, likewise, how coping behaviours and attitudes shape development. The chapter will now turn to the issues of quality of life and well-being in young people with coeliac disease.

Quality of life and psychosocial well-being

Across both epidemiological and clinical studies, children and young people with long-term conditions are known to be at increased risk for psychosocial adjustment problems (Hysing et al., 2009). The daily impact of chronic illness can manifest itself through restrictions in daily activities at home, at school, and with friends, and the affects can be attributed to both illness-specific problems (e.g. symptoms, pain, demanding treatment regimens) and to psychological dimensions (e.g. life threat potential, visibility, intrusiveness) shared across different physical disorders.

Given that the GFD can be difficult for a substantial number of children and young people to accept and follow, and that some report feeling different from their friends, see others as more independent and feel anger in response to having to follow a GFD, several studies have looked at the association between coeliac disease and the GFD and measures of quality of life (QoL) and psychosocial well-being. To date, the results are equivocal. The methodological quality of studies differs with regards to descriptive data that are presented (e.g. time since diagnosis, quality of dietary self-management), the nature of measurements used (e.g. generic versus disease specific measures of QoL), type of comparison sample (e.g. healthy controls, normative sample) and study design. In a robust prospective 10-year follow-up study, van Koppen et al. (2009) found evidence of impaired health-related QoL at diagnosis in young children (aged 2–4 years) who were symptomatic. QoL was significantly improved after one year of the GFD compared to those who had been asymptomatic at diagnosis. Further, at 10-year follow-up, general health-related QoL was reported to be equivalent to those in a general Dutch reference sample, but slightly lower when measured using a coeliac disease-specific QoL measure. The finding of reduced health-related QoL replicates previous findings in children and young people with coeliac disease (van Doorn et al., 2008), and the often found discrepancy between generic and disease specific measures highlights how generic instruments can veil specific difficulties related to particular long-term conditions. In terms of dietary self-management and QoL, young people who are reported to be better at following the dietary recommendations, and those diagnosed before the age of six, have been found to have QoL scores equivalent to healthy controls (Cinquetti et al., 1999).

Overall, despite the potential restrictions that the GFD can place on a child's lifestyle, the evidence seems to suggest that the majority of children, once diagnosed and on a GFD, have comparable QoL to healthy controls; young people with coeliac disease are able to participate in almost all activities at school, with only a minority reporting difficulty in adjusting their lifestyle (Roma et al., 2010). The most important factors identified by children and parents as likely to enhance QoL are better food labelling, improvement in the availability of gluten-free products, and better education about coeliac disease and its treatment.

In terms of psychological difficulties, several studies have suggested poorly defined 'emotional symptoms' as being common among children and young people with coeliac disease, but few studies have investigated the nature and prevalence of specific mental health difficulties. To help address this issue, Pynnonen et al. (2004) in Finland used diagnostic criteria and structured psychiatric interviews to examine the prevalence of symptoms and disorders in a sample of 29 young people with coeliac disease. The results showed significantly higher lifetime prevalence of major depressive disorder (31% versus 7%) and disruptive behaviour disorder (28% versus 3%) in the coeliac disease sample compared to non-coeliac disease matched comparisons. Interestingly, these mental health difficulties preceded the diagnosis of coeliac disease and its treatment, thus indicating the pre-treatment phase as a time of increased risk. The researchers further suggested a possible physiological mechanism underlying the link between coeliac disease and depression, suggesting that some people are more vulnerable to depression when living with untreated coeliac disease. Research has also shown young women with coeliac disease, particularly older adolescents, to be at risk for disordered eating behaviour, and shape and weight concerns (Karwautz et al., 2008).

Overall, the literature is mixed with positive and negative findings in relation to the association between coeliac disease, QoL and psychosocial well-being. While health-related QoL does seem to be impaired by the condition, this is most prominent in the pre-diagnosis and pre-treatment phases and can be improved when following a GFD. A range of emotional symptoms or responses to coeliac disease and the GFD are found across studies, but the more robust ones show an increased risk for lifetime depressive and behavioural disorders, and eating difficulties for women. The task for future research is to tease apart the psychological challenges and responses to coeliac disease and the GFD and link this to developmental risk and protective mechanisms. For clinicians, there is a message about how to listen more closely to the stories from children, young people and families living with coeliac disease, being aware of the above findings, and taking the time to ask the necessary questions and make appropriate adjustments to care and help in the transition to adulthood.

Psychosocial aspects of coeliac disease in adulthood

From a medical perspective the management of coeliac disease is straightforward and effective. For the vast majority of people the treatment is successful, leading to a decrease in reported symptoms, the reversal of gut damage, and the reduction in the long-term risk of serious health conditions such as cancer and osteoporosis. However, the GFD brings with it enormous lifestyle changes for the person managing the condition and their family, particularly in western societies where the diet relies heavily on cereal based foods. These lifestyle changes have been found to lead to psychosocial difficulties for some people with coeliac disease and therefore it is the aim of this section to explore the psychosocial impact of the condition and the GFD on adults.

Diagnosis

At the point of diagnosis the main management strategy prescribed is a strict, lifelong therapeutic GFD. This is achieved with education and support of dietetic and gastroenterology services (Ciclitira et al., 2010). Research has shown that people being diagnosed with coeliac disease may already be experiencing psychological distress as a result of long-term, unexplained symptoms and a longstanding absence of a clear diagnosis prior to this point (Hin et al., 1999; Jones, 2007). Therefore diagnosis can itself result in psychosocial reactions, including relief, anxiety and anger and those with symptoms at the point of diagnosis can have a poorer quality of life (Lohiniemi et al., 1998). At present there are no studies found to consider the psychological consequences of the diagnostic processes themselves.

Management of the Gluten-Free Diet (GFD)

As we have already learned, the GFD requires the person with coeliac disease to remove all gluten-containing foods from their diet. This major change to the person's eating behaviour can lead people to experience anxiety, depression, anger, fatigue and a reduced quality of life, largely due to the restrictions placed on the person (Hallert et al., 1998, 2003; Hauser et al., 2007).

Eating is not only essential but a social pastime. However, once a diet is restricted, this pastime becomes more difficult to manage, especially outside the home. It requires more thought and planning, and not all restaurants cater easily for people on a GFD. The different eating behaviours associated with the diet also bring into focus the fact that the person with coeliac disease is different. For some, this situation can be difficult to manage and can lead to poorer psychological well-being (e.g. Hallert et al., 2003).

The quality of dietary self-management in coeliac disease has been found to be associated with both good and poor psychological well-being. Several research groups in Italy, including groups led by Addolorato and Usai, have considered the association between depression and anxiety and adherence to the GFD. Their findings suggest that on the whole, good dietary self-management leads to lower scores on general anxiety and depression, although this may also be associated with greater social phobia in some people with coeliac disease. However, the picture remains slightly unclear, with other research suggesting a link between good dietary self-management and a *poorer* quality of life, particularly when the person has been following the diet for a number of years (Hallert, 1998, 2003). It is interesting to consider this association, given the importance placed on the GFD from the point of diagnosis. These findings have implications for practice in order to ensure that people who are potentially at risk of a poorer quality of life as a result of conscientious dietary self-management are identified at the point of diagnosis and supported appropriately.

Psychosocial well-being and quality of life

Following a GFD can have positive effects on quality of life, with improvements found within the first year after diagnosis (e.g. Ciacci et al., 2003). However, studies have also identified high state anxiety in people newly diagnosed with coeliac disease, with women being particularly at risk (Addolorato et al., 2008a; Hauser et al., 2010). This tends to reduce during the first year following diagnosis, leading to the conclusion that this is 'reactive anxiety' associated with the diagnosis of a long-term condition (Addolorato et al., 2001). Some researchers have suggested that continued anxiety may be seen in the form of social phobia, lending weight to the notion that the person is seen as socially different due to the changes in their eating behaviours (Ciacci et al., 2003).

This anxiety may be explained somewhat by the person's self efficacy for the GFD, i.e. the extent to which they believe they have the resources to manage the diet. Knowledge drawn from the literature on the dietary management of other long-term conditions suggests that a person's self efficacy for the GFD may change depending on the setting, with people with coeliac disease able to manage the diet well in the home, where food intake can be controlled, but less self-efficacious outside the home, for example in restaurants, at friend's houses or on holiday (e.g. Ciacci et al., 2003; Hallert et al., 2003). This 20-year-old man, diagnosed for one year illustrates the point:

> 'The trouble comes when I go out with others for meals, go to people's houses or go abroad. This can become incredibly embarrassing as I always have to be rude and turn down food, make people go out of their way to find alternatives, or just not eat at all. People often do go out of their way and spend money on special ingredients or chose coeliac-friendly restaurants, but I personally hate that. I just want to be normal and rather than make plans change, I would rather go hungry. Going abroad is simple; I eat peanuts and crisps and nothing else for the duration of the holiday.' (Rose, 2009)

Depression has been found to be associated with coeliac disease both at the point of diagnosis and in those who have been living with the condition for many years, and managing a GFD. In one Italian study the figure was found to be 57% (Addolorato et al., 2001). Studies have further shown that the depression is not only a result of nutritional malabsorption, but a consequence of managing the condition, with those on a GFD more likely to experience more frequent and more severe episodes of depression than those on a normal diet (Siniscalchi et al., 2005). This may also be linked to the presence of social difficulties for the person with coeliac disease, and the challenges associated with managing the diet outside the home, e.g. in restaurants and on holiday. Depression has also been found to be associated with other aspects of poor psychological well-being, including social phobia, poorer quality of life and fatigue (e.g. Addolorato et al., 2008b; Siniscalchi et al., 2005), but research has yet to determine clearly the nature of these associations and their relationship to the GFD.

A number of studies have considered quality of life (QoL) in people living with coeliac disease. These have mostly been conducted in Europe, particularly Finland, and the findings are rather mixed. Some of the studies show an improvement in QoL following diagnosis which supports the notion that people are relieved to finally have a diagnosis for their unexplained symptoms as well as experiencing an improvement in symptoms (Ciacci et al., 2003; Lohiniemi et al., 1998). However, in some studies, the participants were experiencing a reduced QoL and sometimes this was associated with anxiety, depression and managing the GFD (Hallert et al., 2003). Gender also seems to play a part in QoL in people with coeliac disease, with research indicating that women with the condition report experiencing reduced QoL and more gastrointestinal symptoms than men (Hallert et al., 2003), with more symptoms leading to poorer QoL. Men and women also appear to cope with the social aspects of the GFD in different ways (e.g. Hallert et al., 1998, 2003).

Coeliac disease and the GFD have also been found to be associated with other psychosocial consequences, for example anger, which has been linked to poor dietary self-management, and a sense of difference (Ciacci et al., 2002). Anger has also been related to sadness, perhaps as a consequence of being diagnosed with a life-long, incurable condition, notwithstanding the fact that the management of the condition is highly effective (Ciacci et al., 2002). Fatigue is commonly found in people with coeliac disease and is associated with depression (Siniscalchi et al., 2005); however, this can also be a symptom of undiagnosed coeliac disease, especially due to its link with anaemia. It remains unclear whether this is a physiological effect or is related to the burden of the condition and the GFD, which has been found to be greater in women than men. This 48-year-old woman, diagnosed for 14 years sums it up:

> 'Life with coeliac disease can be hard. Even sticking to the diet, I often feel poorly. I struggle with energy levels and often feel drained. I have to really push myself hard to keep going with everyday activities. If I do eat something I shouldn't, it totally wipes me out for a few days and then it takes a good couple of weeks before I'm back to normal. I often feel quite "down" and "insecure" and cry at the slightest of things which I understand is a symptom of the disease. I sometimes feel quite impatient with people, particularly at work, which I recognise as me being tired and which I find difficult to handle.' (Rose, 2009)

Psychosocial intervention

Little published research has considered the area of psychosocial intervention for people with coeliac disease. Although guidelines suggest dietary advice in the form of nutritional counselling, and a multidisciplinary team approach is suggested for the management of coeliac disease (Pietzak, 2005) only one group of Italian researchers has published recent data on the effectiveness of psychological counselling (Addolorato et al., 2004). Their findings suggest that an approach that considers general stress management alongside specific difficulties associated with managing the GFD can lead to a reduction in anxiety and depression over the first six months following diagnosis. This may not be essential for all people diagnosed with condition and may require an initial screening for psychological distress and other risk factors. Here, also, the person's illness perceptions and self efficacy for the gluten-free diet may indicate who would benefit most from interventions of this nature and who does not require it.

Summary

Coeliac disease is becoming more recognized in daily life and more people are being diagnosed, although the presentation of the condition remains complex. The psychosocial picture of coeliac disease is a mixed one. Researchers have identified numerous psychosocial consequences of living with the condition and managing the GFD. However, research of this nature, particularly in the UK, is in its infancy. Further studies are needed to understand why some people cope well with the condition and the diet whilst others struggle. Specifically, researchers need to examine the roles of illness representations and self efficacy and their relationship with psychosocial well-being and dietary self-management, and the viability and effectiveness of psychosocial interventions for those who struggle. As the condition becomes more integrated into daily life, services for people with coeliac disease need to consider not only diagnostic methods and the GFD, but also the psychosocial consequences thereof, integrating psychological thinking into everyday practice, and psychosocial interventions where necessary. This will mirror the multidisciplinary management of many other acute and long-term conditions where a bio-psychosocial approach is the norm.

Further reading

'Special Issue: Evidence-based assessment in pediatric psychology' (2008) *Journal of Pediatric Psychology*, 33(9): 911–1064.

Howdle, P. (2007) *Your Guide to Coeliac Disease*. Royal Society of Medicine.

Petrie, K. and Weinman, J.A. (1997) *Perceptions of Health and Illness*. Harwood Academic Publishers.

Edwards, M. and Titman, P. (2010) *Promoting Psychological Well-being in Children with Acute and Chronic Illness*. Jessica Kingsley.

References

Addolorato, G., Capristo, E., Ghittoni, G., Valeri, C., Mascianà, R., Ancona, C. et al. (2001) 'Anxiety but not depression decreases in coeliac patients after one-year gluten-free diet: A longitudinal study', *Scandinavian Journal of Gastroenterology*, 36(5): 502–6.

Addolorato, G., De Lorenzi, G., Abenavoli, L., Leggio, L., Capristo, E. and Gasbarrini, G. (2004) 'Psychological support counselling improves gluten-free diet compliance in coeliac patients with affective disorder', *Alimentary Pharmacology & Therapeutics*, 20: 777–82.

Addolorato, G., Mirijello, A., D'Angelo, C., Leggio, L., Ferrulli, A., Vonghia, L. et al. (2008a) 'Social phobia in coeliac disease', *Scandinavian Journal of Gastroenterology*, 43: 410–15.

Addolorato, G., Mirijello, A., D'Angelo, C., Leggio, L., Ferrulli, A., Abenavoli, L. et al. (2008b) 'State and trait anxiety and depression in patients affected by gastrointestinal diseases: Psychometric evaluation of 1641 patients referred to an internal medicine outpatient setting', *International Journal of Clinical Practise*, 62: 1063–9.

Anson, O., Weizman, Z. and Zeevi, N. (1990) 'Celiac disease: Parental knowledge and attitudes of dietary compliance', *Pediatrics*, 85: 98–103.

Bandura, A. (1997) *Self Efficacy: The Exercise of Control*. New York: W.H. Freeman.

BSPGHAN (2006) *Guideline for the Diagnosis and Management of Coeliac Disease in Children*.

Ciacci, C., Iavarone, A., Siniscalchi, M., Romano, R. and De Rosa, A. (2002) 'Psychological dimensions of celiac disease: Toward an integrated approach', *Digestive Diseases and Sciences*, 47: 2082–7.

Ciacci, C., D'Agate, C., De Rosa, A., Franzese, C., Errichiello, S., Gasperi, V. et al. (2003) 'Self-rated quality of life in Celiac disease', *Digestive Diseases and Sciences,* 48: 2216–20.

Ciclitira, P.J, Dewar, D.H., McLaughlin, S.D. and Sanders, D.S. (2010) *The Management of Adults with Coeliac Disease.* British Society of Gastroenterology.

Cinquetti, M., Trabucchi, C., Menegazzi, N., Comucci, A., Bressan, F. and Zoppi, G. (1999) 'Psychological problems connected to dietary restrictions in the adolescent with coeliac disease', *Pediatric Med Chir,* 21: 279–83.

Fabiani, E., Taccari, L.M., Ratsch, I.M., Di Giuseppe, S., Coppa, G.V. and Catassi, C. (2000) 'Compliance with gluten free diet in adolescents with screening-detected celiac disease: A 5-year follow-up study', *Journal of Pediatrics,* 136: 841–3.

Feighery, C. (1999) 'Fortnightly review: Coeliac disease', *British Medical Journal,* 319: 236–9.

Gray, A.M. and Papanicolas, I.N. (2010) 'Impact of symptoms on quality of life before and after diagnosis of coeliac disease: Results from a UK population survey', *BMC Health Service Research,* 10: 105–11.

Hagger, M. (2010) 'Health psychology review: Advancing theory and research in health psychology and behavioural medicine', *Health Psychology Review,* 4(1): 1–5.

Hallert, C., Granno, C., Grant, C., Hulten, S., Midhagen, G., Strom, M. et al. (1998) 'Quality of life of adult coeliac patients treated for 10 years', *Scandinavian Journal of Gastroenterology,* 33: 933–8.

Hallert, C., Sandlund, O., and Broqvist, M. (2003) 'Perceptions of health-related quality of life of men and women living with coeliac disease', *Scandinavian Journal of Caring Sciences,* 17: 301–7.

Hauser, W., Stallmach, A., Caspary, W.F. and Stein, J. (2007) 'Predictors of reduced health-related quality of life in adults with coeliac disease', *Alimentary Pharmacology and Therapeutics,* 25: 569–78.

Hauser, W., Janke, K.H., Klump, B., Gregor, M. and Hinz, A. (2010) 'Anxiety and depression in adult patients with celiac disease on a gluten-free diet', *World J Gastroenterol,* 16: 2780–7.

Hin, H., Bird, G., Fisher, P., Mahy, N., Jewell, D. (1999) 'Coeliac disease in primary care: Case finding study', *BMJ,* 16(318): 164–7.

Hopman, E.G.D., le Cessie, S., von Blomberg, B.M.E. and Mearin, M. L. (2006) 'Nutritional management of the gluten-free diet in young people with Celiac Disease in the Netherlands', *Journal of Pediatric Gastroenterology and Nutrition,* 4: 102–8.

Hopper, A.D., Cross, S.S., Hurlstone, D.P., McAlindon, M.E., Lobo, A.J., Hadjivassiliou, M. et al. (2007) 'Pre-endoscopy serological testing for coeliac disease: Evaluation of a clinical decision tool', *British Medical Journal,* 334: 729–34.

Hysing, M., Elgen, I., Gillberg, C. and Lundervold, A.J. (2009) 'Emotional and behavioural problems in subgroups of children with chronic illness: Results from a large scale population study', *Child: Care, Health and Development,* 35(4): 527–33.

Jackson, P.T., Glasgow, J.F.T. and Thom, R. (1985) 'Parents' understanding of coeliac disease and diet', *Archives of Disease of Childhood,* 60: 672–4.

Jones, R. (2007) 'Coeliac disease in primary care', *BMJ,* 7(334): 704–5.

Jones, R., Hunt, C., Stevens, R., Dalrymple, J., Driscoll, R., Sleet, S. and Blanchard Smith, J. (2009) 'Management of common gastrointestinal disorders: Quality criteria based on patients' views and practice guidelines', *British Journal of General Practice*, 59: e199–e208.

Karwautz, A., Wagner, G., Berger, G., Sinnreich, U., Grylli, V. and Huber, W-D. (2008) 'Eating pathology in adolescents with celiac disease', *Psychosomatics*, 49(5): 399–406.

Leventhal, H., Halm, E., Horowitz, C., Leventhal, E.A. and Ozakinci, G. (2005) 'Living with chronic illness: A contextualized, self-regulation approach', in S. Sutton, A. Baum and M. Johnston (eds), *The Sage Handbook of Health Psychology* (pp. 197–240). London: Sage.

Lohiniemi, S., Mustalahti, K., Collin, P., Mäki, M. (1998) 'Measuring quality of life in coeliac disease patients', in S. Lohiniemi, P. Collin, M. Mäki (eds), *Changing Features of Coeliac Disease*, p. 71. Tampere: The Finnish Coeliac Society.

Mearin, M.L. (2007) 'Celiac disease among children and adolescents', *Current Problems in Pediatric and Adolescent Health Care*, 37: 86–105.

NICE (2009) *Coeliac Disease: Recognition and Assessment of Coeliac Disease*. UK: National Institute for Health and Clinical Excellence.

Nouwen, A., Law, G.U., Hussain, S., McGovern, S. and Napier, H. (2009) 'Comparison of the role of self-efficacy and illness representations in relation to dietary self-care and diabetes distress in adolescents with type 1 diabetes', *Psychology and Health*, 24: 1071–84.

Olsson, C., Hornell, A., Ibarsson, A. and Sydner, Y.M. (2008) 'The everyday life of adolescent coealics: Issues of importance for compliance with the gluten-free diet', *Journal of Human Nutrition and Dietetics*, 21: 359–67.

Olsson, C., Lyon, P., Hornell, A., Ivarsson, A. and Sydner, Y.M. (2009) 'Food that makes you different: The stigma experienced by adolescents with celiac disease', *Qualitative Health Research*, 19(7): 976–84.

Pietzak, M.M. (2005) 'Follow-up of patients with coeliac disease: Achieving compliance with treatment', *Gastroenterology*, 128(4): S135–41.

Pynnonen, P.A., Isometsa, E.T., Aronen, E.T., Verkasalo, M.A., Savilahti, E. and Aalberg, V.A. (2004) 'Mental disorders in adolescents with celiac disease', *Psychosomatics*, 45(4): 325–35.

Roma, E., Roubani, A., Kolia, E., Panayiotou, J., Zellos, A. and Syriopoulou, V.P. (2010) 'Dietary compliance and life style of children with coelic disease', *Journal of Human Nutrition and Dietetics*, 23: 176–82.

Rose, C. (2009) *Living with Coeliac Disease*, unpublished MSc thesis, University of Coventry.

Rostrom, A., Murray, J.A. and Kagnoff, M.F. (2006) 'American Gastroenterological Association (AGA) Institute Technical Review on the diagnosis and management of celiac disease', *Gastroenterology*, 131: 1981–2002.

Schmidt, S., Petersen, C. and Bullinger, M. (2003) 'Coping with chronic disease from the perspective of children and adolescents – a conceptual framework and its implications for participation', *Child: Care, Health and Development*, 29(1): 63–75.

Siniscalchi, M., Iovino, P., Tortora, R., Forestiero, S., Somma, A., Cauano, L. et al. (2005) 'Fatigue in adult coeliac disease', *Alimentary Pharmacology & Therapeutics*, 22: 489–94.

Van Doorn, R.K., Winkler, L.M., Zwinderman, K.H., Mearin, M.L. and Koopman, H.M. (2008) 'COELIAC DISEASEDUX: A disease-specific health-related quality of life questionnaire for children with celiac disease', *Pediatric Gastroenterology and Nutrition*, 47(2): 147–52.

Van Koppen, E.J., Schweizer, J.J., Csizmadia, C.G.D.S., Krom, Y., Hylkema, H.B., van Geel, A.M., Koopman, H.K., Verloove-Vanhorick., P. and Mearin, M.L. (2009) 'Long-term health and quality-of-life consequences of mass screening for childhood celiac disease: A 10-year follow-up study', *Pediatrics*, 123(4): e582–8.

Acknowledgements

The authors would like to thank Dr Jan Oyebode, Dr Eleni Theodosi, Kate Rose and Dr Sarah Ford for their contributions to the on-going research at the University of Birmingham which has informed this chapter.

10

Working with Vulnerable People: Experiences of Disability

Mary Larkin

Overview

- Approaches to disability
- The medical model of disability
- The social model of disability
- Inequalities experienced by disabled people
- Health and social care practitioners working with disabled people
- Conclusion

The relationship between long-term conditions and disability is complex; whether or not someone with a long-term condition experiences disability depends on a number of factors such as the pain associated with the condition, the effectiveness of the treatment available, age and onset of the condition, the extent to which a person self identifies as disabled and the social context of disability. Nonetheless, the trajectory of many long-term conditions, such as Cystic Fibrosis, Multiple Sclerosis and Alzheimer's disease results in physical and mental disabilities at some point (Beckett, 2009; Bradby, 2009; Salway et al., 2007). An understanding of the experience of disability in our society and its implications for practice is therefore essential for those working with people with long-term conditions in health and social care.

In order to equip health and social care practitioners to work more effectively with disabled people, this chapter will focus on 'disability' in the broadest sense in terms of physical/mental disabilities which can result in functional and activity limitations. It will consider different approaches to disability in the United Kingdom which have influenced policy and practice, as well as give examples of the relationship between inequality and disability in our society today. In addition, the specific implications for those working with disabled people in health and social care settings will be discussed. During these discussions, reference will be made to the ways in which current changes within the health and social care system affect health and social care practice in relation to disabled people.

Approaches to disability

The fact that many different terms have been used to define disability (Beckett, 2009; Hughes, 1998) indicates that this concept is more of a question of social definition rather than a statement of fact or objective truth. Indeed, there is an extensive body of literature about the social construction of the concept of 'disability' (Oliver, 1990, 1996, 1998). Social construction refers to the way that aspects of society or behaviour are actively 'constructed' as a result of social relations and human agency at particular points in time in particular cultures rather than being 'natural' or biological in origin (Cuff et al., 2006; Giddens, 1992). Consequently, the way disability is constructed has changed over time. The argument that disability is socially constructed is supported by evidence of historical changes in the way people with disabilities have been viewed and the way that such changes have shaped elements of policy (Finkelstein, 1981, Oliver, 1990; Shakespeare, 2006). The 'medical' model of disability and the 'social' model of disability are both examples of these changing constructions.

The medical model of disability

The rise of biomedicine meant that from the nineteenth century disability became medicalized and disabled people were constructed as being medical problems who were dependent on medical care and the medical profession. This approach to disability is called the 'medical' model of disability. It involves the colonization of disability by medicine and is illustrated in Figure 10.1.

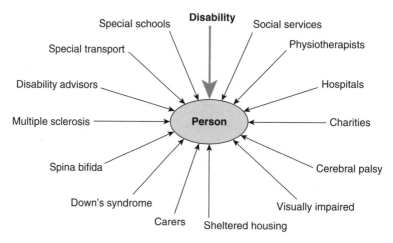

Figure 10.1   The medical model of disability

Source: Larkin, 2011

Within this model, disability is individualized in terms of individual pathology; impairments are classified. Some examples are given in Figure 10.1, such as cerebral palsy and spina bifida. The emphasis is on these being an individual problem and on the impairment rather than the person. Disabled people are also treated as 'patients' and labelled as abnormal. Furthermore, disablement can only be treated by medical intervention. Therefore it is the medical profession and other allied professions (for instance, physiotherapists) who have the power to decide how the person with the disability is treated. Consequently, the medical model leads to disabled people being passive objects of 'intervention, treatment and reha-bilitation' (Oliver, 1990: 50). In addition, they are not involved in decisions that have major implications for their quality of life in that they cannot, for example, determine the extent and quality of their education and whether they can work or not. A final characteristic of this model is its exclusive focus on the association between impairment and disability which means that the role of the environment in which disabled people live is ignored.

The medical model has influenced legislation and policy about the disabled and disability significantly. One of the consequences is that serv-ices and practice have been determined by able-bodied people and have focused on addressing what professionals perceive to be disabled people's requirements and their need for functional rehabilitation. More impor-tantly, the extent to which medicalized views of disability feature in this model has meant the focus within practice has been on individuals' impairments and vulnerabilities rather than the social constraints to social participation for people with disabilities.

Not only does this model ignore the experiential, social and situational components of disability but it also has lifelong and oppressive consequences for disabled people (Hughes, 1998; Hyde, 2006a; Oliver, 1990, 1996). Unsurprisingly, the medical model has been challenged and since the 1990s, there has been a move towards the demedicalization of disability and a new conceptual framework for understanding disability – the social model of disability.

The social model of disability

The social model (see Figure 10.2 below) constructs disability in a radically different way from the medical model. It argues that disability is not caused by an individual's impairment but that it is the attitudinal, cultural, social and environmental constraints imposed by a society geared towards a norm of ablebodiedness that oppresses disabled people and curtails their opportunities and capabilities.

From the 1970s several factors played a significant role in the development of this model of disability. One was the growth in the power of the disability movement; in the 1960s and 1970s there were only organizations *for* disabled people run by able-bodied people. In the 1980s organizations *of* disabled people started to emerge. These are also referred to as user-led organizations and are run exclusively by disabled people. Although they co-exist alongside organizations *for* disabled people, their number and

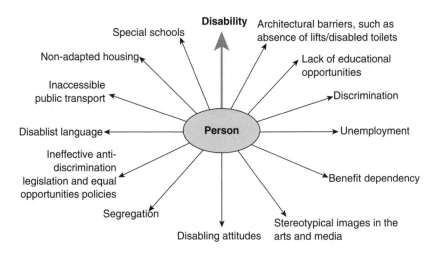

Figure 10.2   The social model of disability

Source: Larkin, 2011

power has increased. As a consequence, the disability movement has developed a high profile political agenda that has challenged dominant discourses about disability, and taken action that has shaped legislation which has promoted the equalization of opportunities for, and integration of, disabled persons into society (Hughes, 1998; Hyde, 2006a). Since the 1990s, the growth of an increasingly influential body of literature written by activists, such as Mike Oliver and Tom Shakespeare, in the disability movement has also contributed to the development of the social model of disability.

The social model of disability concentrates on society and what it does to keep people disabled. Integral to this is the examination of how society needs to change in order to stop disabling people with disabilities and to emancipate them so that they can participate in society and become empowered as citizens with rights. Adoption of the social model has resulted in a distinct set of policies which have aimed to abolish the fixed notion of 'normality' to which disabled people have to aspire and to make the physical, cultural and economic environment accessible and less discriminatory for people with disabilities. Consequently, there have been changes such as ramps and chairlifts, and equal opportunities policies. There have also been policies introduced in an attempt to alleviate the oppression of disabled people. Examples are the legislation in the 1970s and 1980s to reclassify people once regarded as 'idiots', 'mongols', 'retarded' and so forth. In addition, there have been policies to involve them in decision-making about their own lives, integrate them into ordinary life, and enable them to live independently as possible (Fawcett, 2000; Hyde, 2006b; Oliver, 1990, 2004).

This change in approach to disability has been viewed positively because it has led to the greater empowerment of disabled people, reduced discrimination against them and increased their opportunities, independence and integration into society. However, it has been criticized for focusing solely on disability in terms of social discrimination and social oppression, and for not acknowledging the way that bodily impairment can impact on disabled people's ability to engage in everyday life as much as say, discrimination. Recent criticisms have also been made about the way that the social model of disability does not engage with the breadth of experience that 'disability' has been shown to encompass (Hyde, 2006a; Oliver, 2004; Twigg, 2006). Furthermore, despite changes in policy that occurred as a result of the adoption of this model, health and social care practice has remained paternalistic. This includes the continuation of the professional definition of need and level of service, and an approach to disabled people based on working 'for' rather than alongside them. In addition, disability has not been completely demedicalized, mainly because of the ongoing power of the medical profession over the lives of disabled people (Foster et al., 2006; Glasby, 2010).

Inequalities experienced by disabled people

The body of literature about disability referred to above has provided many insights into the life experiences of disabled people. Academic research has made a considerable contribution; articles about disability regularly appear in social policy, social work, and health and social care journals. In addition there are now some well established national and international journals which focus exclusively on disability issues. One of these is *Disability and Society* which was founded in 1986. There are also University disability research units, such as those at The University of Leeds and Lancaster University. Other research about disability and disabled people has been carried out and/or funded by government departments and charities (such as Arthritis Research UK and the Multiple Sclerosis Society). The emphasis in the research carried out on the importance of the voices of the participants has shown that the move to the social model of disability has improved the lives of disabled people. However, it has also highlighted the many inequalities, such as reduced educational opportunities and income levels, that they still experience.

When working with disabled people, health and social care practitioners need to be aware of these sorts of inequalities. Some examples that have been identified in the aforementioned research and the way that they constitute barriers to the social inclusion of disabled people in our society are as follows:

- **Prejudice and discrimination:** Prejudice and discrimination against people who happen to be disabled is still common and negatively affects many areas of their lives. It has been argued that amongst the most notable causes are professionals' disabling attitudes (Foster et al., 2006). There is also evidence that more subtle forms of prejudice exist in the mass media. For instance, the absence of images of disabled people taking part in everyday life, such as working and playing an active role in their families, has led to negative views of the extent of their capabilities (Deal, 2007; Wates, 2004). The inevitable internalization of such stereotyping can cause much distress for disabled people; a Norwegian study by Grue and Laerum (2002) of physically disabled mothers found that they felt constant pressure to show that they were managing 'normally' and feared that their children would be taken from them if they did not appear to live up to societal expectations of being an 'ordinary' mother.
- **Employment:** Whilst many disabled people want to work, getting suitable jobs remains problematic despite legislation designed to improve their chances of high rates of employment. Figures show that they are about twice as likely to be unemployed

than non-disabled people. When they are in paid employment they are also more likely to do part-time work which generally has lower status and pay, less job security and fewer employment rights (Bailey, 2004; Bambra et al., 2005). Furthermore, they face many disadvantages in terms of career progression (Sayce, 2009).

- **Health and social care**: People with a disability experience barriers when accessing health care. These barriers include health professionals' discriminatory attitudes, lack of knowledge and understanding of their health issues, delays in receiving services and inconsistencies in service delivery. There is also much evidence that those who live in the community do not receive adequate social care because of the failure of community services to respond to their needs adequately (Gulliford and Morgan, 2003; Melville, 2005; Slade et al., 2009).
- **Education**: Studies have shown that people who are disabled are disadvantaged throughout the education system. Consequently they are far more likely to have lower or no academic qualifications than non-disabled people (Disability Rights Commission, 2006; Hyde, 2006b; Smith and Twomey, 2002).
- **Income**: Disabled people are the largest group in receipt of benefits in the United Kingdom – they account for about 25% of benefit expenditure. Benefit dependency invariably means living on a low income and being at greater risk of poverty. Indeed, it is estimated that 45% of disabled adults live in poverty (Bambra et al., 2005; Hyde, 2006b).
- **Housing**: Although many disabled people live in their own homes, they still face considerable disadvantages in relation to housing. Choice is limited when it comes to meeting their housing needs. They are also more likely to live in public housing and less likely to rent privately or have a mortgage than non-disabled people (Stevens, 2004). Another study showed how disabled people with mobility problems are often excluded from the owner occupation market. This is because the design of houses for owner occupation frequently renders them unsuitable for their needs (Thomas, 2004).
- **Social and personal life**: Disabled people have fewer interpersonal relationships than non-disabled people and this is reflected in the fact that, overall, disabled people are less likely to have the opportunity to have sexual relationships and to have children (O' Grady et al., 2004).

Health and social care practitioners working with disabled people

The debate about models of disability has many implications for professional and inter-professional practice in health and social care with disabled people, whether it is in a hospital or community setting, both now and in future. With reference to current practice:

- The different approaches to disability and the ensuing policies means that health and social care practitioners need a clear understanding of dominant approaches to disability and the continuing hegemony of features of the medical model

- It is important that health and social care practitioners develop a critical awareness of how polices can shape their work with disabled people and do not refrain from challenging practice if necessary. The use of relevant research can contribute significantly to this critical awareness
- The involvement and empowerment of people with disabilities should be central to practice at all times
- Health and social care practitioners must be sensitive to the ongoing inequalities that people with disabilities experience

When working with disabled people in health and social care settings over the next few years, practitioners will be implementing the huge changes that the health and social care system is currently undergoing as a result of personalization. This new agenda is the main driver behind the development of a variety of initiatives and models in health and social care which aim to increase service users' choice, control and independence so that they 'will be empowered to shape their own lives and the services they receive in all care settings' (Department of Health, 2008a). Those that will have the most significant impact on people who have disabilities are the personalized models of care that have been introduced. These place the individual at the heart of the health and social care process, foster independence in service users as well as giving them more choice and control over the care they receive (Browning, 2007; Glendinning et al., 2009).

As self-directed support is central to these personalized models of care, it is important that health and social care practitioners understand the different forms of such support. One example is *direct payments*. These are cash payments made to individuals assessed as needing services in lieu of social service provision so that they can decide how their care is delivered and buy their support accordingly (Department of Health, 2008b). Another example is the *In Control* model for social care whereby funds are directly allocated to the individuals concerned at the start of the support process. This is to enable the person needing support, as opposed to professionals, to control and to decide how best to use the funds directly allocated to them to meet their needs, live their lives and achieve their goals. *In Control's* self-directed support model includes person centred planning, and examples of the latter are Personal Budgets and Resource Allocation Systems. The intention is that all those receiving adult social care will receive a Personal Budget by 2013 (Department of Health, 2010). Personal Budgets represent both an extension of and development from Direct Payments in that they combine several funding streams in order to enable service users to purchase a much wider variety of support options, such as gym membership or payment to relatives and friends for their help. They also provide service users with the option of choosing services directly provided by their Local Authority or to use a mixture of different services and purchase their own support as well as making their own arrangements.

The mainstreaming of personalized models throughout social care has cross party support and continues at a pace. The move to increased personalization and control is now extending beyond adult social care into health care; personal health budgets are being piloted and *In Control* is branching out into health, education and employment (Edwards and Waters, 2009; Hatton et al., 2008). This transformation of adult health and social care requires complex cultural, structural and procedural adjustments that are predicted to take several years to effect and which impact at organizational and personal levels. Studies have identified some of the issues for service users, exploring the outcomes for different groups of service users across a number of life domains (Glendinning et al., 2008; Henwood and Hudson, 2009). Positive outcomes for users were feelings of being in more control of their lives and improvements in health, quality of life, and levels of community participation (Commission for Social Care Inspection, 2008, 2009; Edwards and Waters, 2009; Waters and Hay, 2009). The case study below is about a lady with disabilities who was allocated a Personal Budget. Although it focuses on one particular type of self-directed support, it illustrates some of the positive outcomes of the move to personalized models within social care. However, such resources are only an option for those who meet the increasingly restrictive eligibility criteria. Outcomes also vary between user groups and depended on their support networks and the extent to which some practitioners exert control over their decision making. Furthermore, responding effectively to some groups, such as those with complex needs, has proved to be more problematic (Browning, 2007; Glynn et al., 2008; Hatton et al., 2008).

How Mary used her personal budget

Mary has Parkinson's disease which affects her physical functioning and cognitive abilities. She uses a wheelchair and requires assistance with moving around. Her husband, James, managed Mary's care without support for a number of years. However, over time, Mary's condition has become much more severe and she has been unable to cope without support. Initially services were provided by morning and evening visits from carers, but this did not work because it was impossible to specify when Mary needed help. Although they dreaded the thought of being parted, Mary and her husband began to think that the only solution was residential care. During the course of trying to avoid residential care they requested advice about a Personal Budget. This enabled Mary to employ a

---

(Continued)

24 hour live in carer who could provide support to Mary in her own home and reduce her husband's caring responsibilities. The carer has now been employed, lives in what was the spare bedroom and the arrangement is working well. Mary feels that because she is in receipt of a Personal Budget and can use it in this way, she has remained independent and in control of her life.
(Adapted from Peak and Walters, 2008)

Practitioners will need to ensure that they are fully informed about the rapid changes that are taking place throughout health and social care as a result of personalization and how these relate to service users who are disabled because of their long-term conditions. Current research indicates that practice varies and that individual practitioners still exert control over the decision making process. This is partly due to constraints imposed by the 'organisational context and broader service environment' (Foster et al., 2006: 125) and some of the inherent complexities and contradictions within frontline practice when implementing personalized social care for people with disabilities. The emerging evidence has identified several ways that practitioners can make empowerment, choice, control and greater equality a reality for these service users. One is that they need to avail themselves of training opportunities about specific aspects of these changes, for example, the move to self assessment and self-directed support as well as changes to the nature of the workforce. They also need to adopt a different approach to their working relationships with disabled people in all settings so that they gain a full understanding of the nature of the condition, properly assess their individual needs, whatever the degree of complexity of these needs, and enable them to take ownership of their support. Whilst working *with* disabled people, practitioners should also work in partnership with each other and other agencies to ensure services are integrated and risks are managed adequately (Hope, 2010; Manthorpe et al., 2009: Redley, 2009).

Conclusion

The evidence and arguments presented in this chapter show that there have been improvements in the lives of people with disabilities but that they continue to experience exclusion and inequalities because of the disabling nature of our society. As health and social care is integral to being disabled, part of securing the continuation of such improvements means that practitioners have a responsibility to challenge complacency in health and social care policy and practice. Integral to this is critical use of current and future policy developments to maximize their potential for the involvement and empowerment of disabled people to ensure they have real choice over the care and services they receive.

Summary

To give health and social care practitioners an understanding of the needs of those who have a disability as a result of a long-term condition, this chapter has focused on the experiences of disabled people in our society in general. In so doing, it has demonstrated how the construction of disability has changed over time, how different constructions shape policy and practice and, most importantly, impacted on the lives of disabled people. Despite more recent moves to empower disabled people, it is clear from research undertaken that they still experience many inequalities. The chapter concluded that in order to effectively contribute to the reduction in these inequalities, practitioners working in health and social care settings need to focus on both challenging and using existing and future policies to obtain the best possible outcomes for people with disabilities.

Further reading

Foster, M., Harris, J., Jackson, K., Morgan, H. and Glendinning, C. (2006) 'Personalised social care for adults with disabilities: a problematic concept for frontline practice', *Health and Social Care in the Community*, 14(2): 125–35.

Oliver, M. (1998) *Disabled People and Social Policy: From Exclusion to Inclusion*. London: Longman.

Oliver, M. (2004) 'If I had a hammer: The social model in action' in J. Swain, S. French, C. Barnes and C. Thomas (eds), *Disabling Barriers, Enabling Environments*. London: Sage in association with the Open University.

References

Bailey, N. (2004) 'Does work pay? Employment, poverty and exclusion from social relations' in C. Pantazis, D. Gordon and R. Levitas (eds), *Poverty and Social Exclusion in Britain. The Millennium Survey*. Bristol: The Policy Press.

Bambra, C., Whitehead, M. and Hamilton, V. (2005) 'Does "welfare-to-work" work? A systematic review of the effectiveness of the UK's welfare-to-work programmes for people with a disability or chronic illness', *Social Science and Medicine*, 60(9): 1905–18.

Beckett, C. (2009) *Human Growth and Development*, 7th edn. London: Sage.

Bradby, H. (2009) *Medical Sociology: An Introduction*. London: Sage.

Browning, D. (2007) *Evaluation of the Self-directed Support Network. A Review of Progress up to 31st March 2007*. London: *in Control* Publications.

Commission for Social Care Inspection (2008) *The State of Social Care in England 2006–07*. London: CSCI.

Commission for Social Care Inspection (2009) *The State of Social Care in England 2007–08*. London: CSCI.

Cuff, E.C., Sharrock, W.W. and Francis, D.W. (2006) *Perspectives in Sociology*, 5th edn. London: Routledge.

Deal, M. (2007) 'Aversive disablism: Subtle prejudice towards disabled people', *Disability and Society*, 22(1): 93–107.

Department of Health (2008a) *An Introduction to Personalisation* [Online]. Available at: www.dh.gov.uk

Department of Health (2008b) *An Introduction to Direct Payments* [Online]. Available at: www.dh.gov.uk

Department of Health (2010) *A Vision for Adult Social Care: Capable Communities and Active Citizens* [Online]. Available at: www.dh.gov.uk

Disability Rights Commission (2006) *Disability Briefing*. Disability Rights Commission Research Paper.

Edwards, T. and Waters, J. (2009). *It's Your Life – Take Control. The Implementation of Self-directed Support in Hertfordshire*. Hertfordshire: Hertfordshire County Council and *in Control* Partnerships.

Fawcett, B. (2000) *Feminist Perspectives on Disability*. England: Pearson Education Limited.

Finkelstein, V. (1981) 'Disability and the helper/helped relationship: An historical view' in A. Brechin, P. Liddiard and J. Swain (eds), *Handicap in a Social World*. London: Hodder and Stoughton.

Foster, M., Harris, J., Jackson, K., Morgan, H. and Glendinning, C. (2006) 'Personalised social care for adults with disabilities: A problematic concept for frontline practice', *Health and Social Care in the Community*, 14(2): 125–35.

Giddens, A. (1992) *The Consequences of Modernity*. Cambridge: Polity Press.

Glasby, J. (2010) 'Personalised public services could revolutionise welfare', *The Guardian*, 7 July. [Online] Available at: http://www.guardian.co.uk/commentis-free/2010/jul/07/public-service-policy-welfare-support

Glendinning, C., Challis, D., Fernandez, J., Jacobs, S., Jones, K., Knapp, M., Manthorpe, G., Moran, N., Netten, A., Stevens, M. and Wilberforce, M. (2008) *Evaluation of the Individual Budgets Pilot Programme: Final Report*. York: Social Policy Research Unit.

Glendinning, C., Arksey, H., Jon, K., Moran, N., Netten, A. and Rabiee, P. (2009) *The Individual Budgets Pilot Projects: Impact and Outcomes for Carers*. York: Social Policy Research Unit.

Glynn, M., Beresford, P., Bewley, C., Branfield, F., Butt, J., Croft, S., Dattani Pitt, K., Fleming, J., Flynn, R., Parmore, C., Postle, K. and Turner, M. (2008) *Person-centred Support: What Service Users and Practitioners Say*. York: Joseph Rowntree Foundation.

Grue, L. and Laerum, K.T. (2002) '"Doing motherhood": Some experiences of mothers with physical disabilities', *Disability and Society*, 17(6): 671–83.

Gulliford, M. and Morgan, M. (eds) (2003) *Access to Health Care*. London: Routledge.

Hatton, C., Duffy, S., Waters, J., Senker, J., Crosby, N., Poll, C., Tyson, A., Towell, D. and O'Brien, J. (2008) *An Evaluation of and Report on in Control's Work 2005–2007*. London: *in Control* Publications.

Henwood, M. and Hudson, B. (2009). *Keeping it Personal: Supporting People with Multiple and Complex Needs. A Report to the Commission for Social Care Inspection*. London: Commission for Social Care Inspection.

Hope, P. (2010) 'Integrated, preventive services are key for people with learning disabilities and the elderly', *Community Care*, 3 February.

Hughes, G. (1998) 'A suitable case for treatment? Constructions of disability' in E. Saraga (ed.), *Embodying the Social: Constructions of Difference*. London: Routledge.

Hyde, M. (2006a) 'Disability' in G. Payne (ed.), *Social Divisions*, 2nd edn. Basingstoke: Macmillan.

Hyde, M. (2000b) 'From welfare-to-work? Social policy for disabled people of working age in the United Kingdom in the 1990s', *Disability and Society*, 15(2): 327–41.

Larkin, M. (2011) *Social Aspects of Health, Illness and Healthcare: A Handbook*. London: McGraw-Hill.

Manthorpe, J., Stevens, M., Rapaport, J., Harris, J., Jacobs, S., Challis, D., Netten, A., Knapp, M., Wilberforce, M. and Glendinning, C. (2009) 'Safeguarding and system change: Early perceptions of the implications for adult protection services of the English individual budgets pilots—a qualitative study', *British Journal of Social Work*, 39(8): 1465–80.

Melville, C. (2005) 'Discrimination and health inequalities experienced by disabled people', *Medical Education*, 39(2): 124–6.

O'Grady, A., Pleasence, P., Balmer, N.J., Buck, A. and Genn, H. (2004) 'Disability, social exclusion and the consequential experience of justiciable problems', *Disability and Society*, 19(4): 259–71.

Oliver, M. (1990) *The Politics of Disablement*. Basingstoke: Macmillan.

Oliver, M. (1996) *Understanding Disability: From Theory to Practice*. Basingstoke: Macmillan.

Oliver, M. (1998) *Disabled People and Social Policy: From Exclusion to Inclusion*. London: Longman.

Oliver, M. (2004) 'If I had a hammer: The social model in action', in J. Swain, S. French, C. Barnes and C. Thomas (eds), *Disabling Barriers, Enabling Environments*. London: Sage in association with the Open University.

Peak, M. and Walters, J. (2008) *My Budget, My Choice*. London: City of London and *in Control* Partnerships.

Redley, M. (2009) 'Understanding the social exclusion and stalled welfare of citizens with learning disabilities', *Disability and Society*, 24(4): 489–50.

Salway, S., Platt, L., Harriss, K. and Chowbey, P. (2007) 'Long-term conditions and Disability Living Allowance: Exploring ethnic differences and similarities in access', *Sociology of Health and Illness*, 29(6): 907–30.

Sayce, L. (2009) *Doing Seniority Differently: A Study of High Fliers Living with Ill-health, Injury or Disability*. London: RADAR.

Shakespeare, T. (2006) *Disability Rights and Wrongs*. Abingdon: Routledge.

Slade, Z., Coulter, A. and Joyce, L. (2009) *Parental Experience of Services for Disabled Children. Qualitative Research.* London: Department for Children, Schools and Families.

Smith, A. and Twomey, B. (2002) 'Labour market experiences of people with disabilities', *Labour Market Trends*, 110(8): 415–27.

Stevens, A. (2004) 'Closer to home: a critique of British Government policy towards accommodating learning disabled people in their own homes', *Critical Social Policy*, 24(2) 233–54.

Thomas, P. (2004) 'The experience of disabled people as customers in the owner occupation market', *Housing Studies*, 19(5): 781–94.

Twigg, J. (2006) *The Body in Health and Social Care.* Basingstoke: Palgrave Macmillan.

Waters, J. and Hay, M. (2009) *Steering my Own Course. The Introduction of Self-directed Support in Cambridgeshire.* Cambridgeshire: Cambridgeshire County Council and *in Control* Partnerships.

Wates, M. (2004) 'Righting the family picture: Disability and family life', in J. Swain, S. French, C. Barnes and C. Thomas (eds), *Disabling Barriers, Enabling Environments.* London: Sage in association with the Open University.

DELIVERING HEALTH AND SOCIAL CARE FOR PEOPLE WITH LONG-TERM CONDITIONS

Introduction

Alistair Hewison

This section includes a series of chapters which examine care provision in the context of policy; the epidemiology of long-term conditions (LTCs); perceptions and assessment of risk; the role of carers in supporting people with LTCs; and the ethical challenges that arise when caring for people with LTCs. These all combine to demonstrate the range of issues that need to be considered when *Delivering health and social care for people with long-term conditions.*

The World Health Organization recommends comprehensive and integrated action to prevent and control chronic diseases (long-term conditions), involving a combination of population wide approaches to reduce risks, and strategies that target individuals at high risk or with established disease. However, ensuring that health and social care services can deliver this system-wide action, whilst maintaining a focus on meeting complex individual needs, presents significant political and organizational challenges. For example political decisions about the allocation of resources have a direct impact on the quality and quantity of care that can be provided. 'Comprehensive and integrated action' is unlikely if funding to support it is lacking. Moreover, if the specific needs of people with one or more long-term condition are to be met, then health and social care organizations must work together, or indeed new organizations may need to be created which are better suited, to work with individuals whose needs do not fit neatly into existing categories of care. There can be confusion over which organization is responsible for which aspect of the person's care, and uncertainty as to what is regarded as a health or social need can result in delays in care being provided. In addition the people delivering services and working with people with LTCs need a broad range of skills and knowledge if they are to 'target individuals at high risk or with established disease'.

In Chapter 11 by Alistair Hewison, 'Delivering health and social care for people with long-term conditions: The policy context', English health care is discussed to demonstrate how the provision of services for people with LTCs is being managed at the macro, meso and micro levels of policy. System changes built around the NHS Social Care Model and the case management approach are evaluated to reveal a mixed picture in terms of successful achievement of stated policy aims. For those seeking to understand the context of care for people with LTCs critical review of policy development in this area is necessary. The rapid pace of change in health and social care and recent proposals to review the funding mechanisms for long-term care, only serve to emphasize this need further. This discussion of the complex policy milieu that shapes the delivery of health and social care for people with LTCs sets the scene for the subsequent chapters which analyse a number of related issues. For example, Chapter 12 by Erica Richardson, 'International experience of integrating health and social care of people living with HIV', takes an international view of the health and social care needs of people living with HIV/AIDS focusing on the different priorities faced in countries of the South, where it remains an infectious disease, and those in the richer countries of the North where it has been 'reframed' as a long-term condition. The integration of health and social care is explored through the use of vignettes and the implications this presents for policy in other countries are discussed.

The following chapter by Tom Heller, 'Worth a risk? Risk taking and people with long-term conditions', examines the significance of the concepts of 'risk' and 'labelling' when considering the needs of people with LTCs. In Chapter 13 the inherent tensions involved in assessing and managing risk are analysed. The dilemma of balancing individual and collective concerns, acceptable and unacceptable risk, and professional versus client notions of risk are explored to demonstrate that risk assessment reflects the power differential between the service user and provider. The nature of LTCs means that those experiencing them will require help and support from those often termed as 'informal carers'. In Chapter 14 by Mary Larkin, 'What about the carers?', the initiatives introduced in England over the past ten years aimed at raising the profile of carers are reviewed. Although caring can be a rewarding experience, it generally has a negative effect on carers' health, income and social life. Given the emphasis in current policy on engaging clients and their carers, as partners in the planning and delivery of services it is important to consider what support is needed to achieve this and whether it is sustainable as the number of people with LTCs increases during the next decade and beyond.

It is clear, even from this brief summary of the chapters in this section, that many ethical questions arise when the care of people with LTCs is discussed in a broader societal context, and this is the focus of the final chapter by Stephen Pattison, 'Ethics and long-term conditions: A reflective approach'. Stephen poses a number of questions including: are there ways that people can prepare themselves in case they develop a long-term condition in the future? Using a personal story to illustrate his questions, he describes a set of values and virtues that may be helpful when faced with experiencing a challenging long-term condition. He argues that these should be set against those broader societal values which often ignore and marginalise the experiences and needs of people living with long-term conditions. He asks is there anything that we could do as a society to help people think about the virtues and values that they might need if they develop a long-term condition themselves?

For some time now it has been recognized that LTCs pose a major policy challenge and that new modes of thinking are needed if effective care is to be provided for people with lifelong illnesses. The material presented in this book records how these 'new modes of thinking' have developed and the effect they have had on care, however the WHO briefing note referred to earlier indicates there is still some way to go before effective care is available for all those who need it. The chapters in Section 3 highlight some of the enduring concerns that need to be addressed if this is to be achieved.

11

Delivering Health and Social Care for People with Long-term Conditions: The Policy Context

Alistair Hewison

Overview

- The number of people with one or more long-term conditions is increasing
- This represents a significant policy challenge for service delivery and organization
- The NHS Social Care Model for long-term conditions in England has been influenced by US approaches and the reform process in the UK
- The policy process is complex and shapes the care people receive

Sixty percent of all deaths in the world are as a result of chronic or long-term conditions, and in Europe this figure rises to 86% (WHO, 2005). There are currently 15.4 million people in England with a Long-term Condition (LTC), and it is estimated that by 2025 there will be 42% more people aged 65 and over, who are therefore at greater risk of developing a LTC, living in England alone. This means the number of people with at least one LTC will rise to 18 million (DH, 2010a). People with LTCs account for a significant and growing proportion of health and social care resources and the costs of their treatment and care amount to nearly £7 in every £10 of health spending in England (DH, 2010a). In order to meet this increased demand for services, the management of LTCs is a key priority for the Department of

Health (DH), the NHS and social care services (DH, 2009a). Encouraging self-care for people with LTCs forms a foundation of this policy response (DH, 2009a). In the light of this situation the purpose of this chapter is to examine the policy shaping services for people with LTCs. Most health care systems in the developed world are designed primarily for treating acute, episodic illness (CHSRF, 2005), and so LTCs represent one of the most important health policy problems facing many countries (Singh, 2008). To address this challenge, changes to the organization and delivery of care for people with LTCs are being made, however there is no evidence to suggest that one policy approach is better than another in this area (Singh, 2008). Furthermore, the wider context the health and social care system is part of, influences the way such policy is developed. This will be demonstrated through examination of the policy response in England, as an example of how a range of factors combine to shape the policy framework in a given setting. First, though there is a need to present a working definition of policy as a starting point for the discussion.

Policy

Policy is not a specific, or concrete concept and so defining it is problematic (Crinson, 2009). Policies are on-going, dynamic, subject to change and involve a course of action or a web of decisions rather than arising from a single decision (Crinson, 2009; Ham and Hill, 1993). Policy making is complex because it can cross national borders, be made by individuals, organizations, agencies and governments and operate at regional, national and international levels (Earle, 2007). In response to this complexity analysts have suggested using a 'stages model' which characterizes policy as a process. An example is presented by Dunn (2004), who outlines eight stages, which are:

1 Agenda setting
2 Policy formulation
3 Policy adoption
4 Policy implementation
5 Policy assessment
6 Policy adaptation
7 Policy succession
8 Policy termination

The purpose of such models is to identify the different phases of the policy process and make it clearer. If policy analysis is concerned with understanding and explaining the substance of policy content, policy decisions and the way decisions are made (Barrett and Fudge, 1981), and it is not possible to encapsulate the nature of policy in a single definition, then breaking it down into a series of stages can help. For example the broad policy agenda is informed by the government's ideological approach. If it is committed to the discipline of the market as a means of governance, often associated with parties on the political 'right', its policies will be different from those on the 'left', which may favour a more collective orientation to societal problems. This also informs the identification of problems/issues. In the case of LTCs, is the demand for care an individual problem (it is each individual's responsibility to provide the means for their own care?) or a state problem (is it a collective responsibility to fund and provide care for anyone who needs it?). The consideration and selection of options for action then follow from the first two stages and so on. The 'stagist' model is helpful in presenting a broad picture of the process (Dorey, 2005); however policy is seldom developed in such a planned, ordered way, and is generally reactive and incremental (Lindblom, 1959, 1979). It is not a rational, objective, neutral activity devoid of values or the play of power (Hunter, 2003) and is often characterized by ambiguity of intent, unpredictability of response, and is complex and problematic (Bergen and While, 2005). Given this complexity, and the absence of a single agreed means of analysing it, an alternative approach is taken here using a model which focuses on the levels of policy making (Hudson and Lowe, 2004) to examine the context of service provision for people with LTCs.

- The macro-level encompasses the broad forces that shape policy such as globalization, the global market place, the rising number of people with LTCs internationally.
- The meso-level is the practice of policy making and the system-wide processes and changes necessary for implementation.
- The micro-level focuses down onto the engagement between consumers and agencies.

This provides a framework for thinking about policy which emphasizes the role of government, health and social care organizations, and individuals in shaping and implementing policy. It is consistent with recent work (Singh, 2008) which found that policy interventions in relation to LTCs generally fall into three categories, which mirror the policy levels identified by Hudson and Lowe (2004).

- System-wide or population health approaches (macro). These focus on developing national policy, structures and the resources needed for major change. They often incorporate an emphasis on disease prevention and health promotion and are designed to operate across settings and providers.
- Health delivery systems or selected components (meso). Health delivery systems use information systems, new roles, and organizational re-design to target the significant components of care. They aim to reduce duplication and improve health outcomes.
- The level of individuals (micro). Initiatives focused on individuals include behavioural change and simple case management. (Singh, 2008)

These interventions, operating at the different levels of policy, are not mutually exclusive and are often used together as part of an overall strategy designed to be appropriate to a specific context (Singh, 2008). This provides a comprehensive yet straightforward framework for examining English policy in the area of LTCs.

English policy for long-term conditions

System-wide approaches: Commissioning services for people with long-term conditions

The Labour government, which came to power in 1997, embarked on a programme of system reform and increased spending on the NHS. Between 2000 and 2007 health spending grew from 5.4% of national income in 1998/9 to 7.2% in 2005/6, and accounted for almost 40% of the increase in public expenditure as a share of national income (Chote, 2007). This was accompanied by widespread system reform aimed at introducing more competitive challenge, or contestability, to NHS providers to reduce waiting times and improve quality (Dixon, 2007). The main elements of this system level policy reform are summarized in Figure 11.1.

Central to the drive to bring about change in service provision and delivery is the commissioning process. In England commissioning is

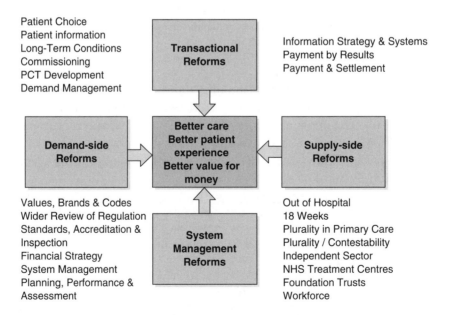

Figure 11.1   System-wide policy reform

Source: adapted from Prime Minister's Strategy Unit (2006)

undertaken by Primary Care Trusts (PCTs) and other public sector commissioners on the 'demand side' to ensure providers deliver the services needed by the local population. Currently PCTs have responsibility for the implementation of health policy and hold a budget for the primary and secondary care needs of their residents (between 200,000 and 1 million people). This has been developed recently into 'World Class Commissioning' which is a national programme to improve health outcomes, reduce health inequalities and increase quality of life (DH, 2010a). The commissioning cycle is made up of eight elements:

1 Assess needs
2 Review current service provision
3 Decide priorities
4 Design service
5 Shape structure of supply
6 Manage demand and ensure appropriate access to care
7 Clinical decision making
8 Managing performance

Each of these elements involves a wide range of activity, for example assessing needs includes measuring disease prevalence, demographics, deprivation levels, the socio-economic make-up and mortality rates of the population in the PCT area. This is followed by a review of current provision to determine which services are already available to meet the needs of people with LTCs and their suitability. These first two phases could result in a particular LTC being chosen as a priority, if a gap in service provision was discovered, for example. Priorities may also be set for improving the health of the LTC population by offering personalized care planning. Services should then be designed to meet the holistic needs of people with LTCs with an emphasis on supporting self-care, delivered by capable provider organizations. The PCT, or other commissioning organization, pay the provider for the delivery of these services. Managing the structure, demand and clinical decision making are all part of the process of providing the service to ensure that improvements are made year on year and clinical and cost effectiveness are achieved. Quality, performance and outcomes are monitored by assessment against metrics or standards written in to the contracts with providers which relate to national and local targets for the care of people with LTCs (DH, 2010a).

When considered in this way the approach seems clear and it might be anticipated that the policy challenge of organizing services to meet the needs of people with LTCs would be met. However, this is just one strand of policy which can conflict with others (de Silva and Fahey, 2008). For example, the focus of the NHS Health and Social Care Model is on pre-vention, supporting self-management and partnership working. However the 'Payment by Results' system, introduced to ensure providers work effi-ciently and economically, may inhibit a change to more community-based care, because it is not in the hospital's financial interest if more people are cared for in the community. The more in-patients treated the more income the hospital receives, a particular concern for 'Foundation Trusts' (de Silva and Fahey, 2008). In this way aspects of policy can conflict and hamper the development of new ways of working in one or more areas. Similar prob-lems can also occur at the next level of policy activity.

Health delivery systems: The NHS and Social Care Long-term Conditions Model

The system structure which shapes the way services for people with LTCs are organized in England is the NHS and Social Care Long-term Conditions Model, which is based on system approaches used in the United States such as the Kaiser Permanente 'pyramid of care' and the Evercare model (Department of Health, 2004). Kaiser Permanente is a not-for-profit health maintenance organization in the United States which is funded through individual and corporate health insurance schemes and integrates prevention, treatment and care. It aims to main-tain its members in good health and avoid inappropriate admissions to hospital by prioritizing the prevention of illness, and treating patients with common conditions. If an unplanned hospital admission occurs it is regarded as a failure in the system. People with LTCs receive struc-tured care from multidisciplinary teams located in the community, based in facilities that are similar to the surgeries used by primary health care teams in the UK, although they are bigger as they house facilities for core diagnostic services and a wider range of staff (Ham, 2005). The Kaiser triangle is used to 'segment' the population of patients with long-term conditions into three groups reflecting their care needs (see Figure 11.2). Several 'Beacon Sites'[1] have been estab-lished in England and have resulted in improvements to the services provided for patients (Ham, 2010). The key elements of this system are summarized below:

- Level 3: Case management – requires the identification of the high intensity users of unplanned secondary care. Care for these patients is co-ordinated by a com-munity matron or other professional(s) using a case management approach, to co-ordinate health and social care.
- Level 2: Disease-specific care management – this involves providing people who have a complex single need or multiple conditions with responsive, specialist

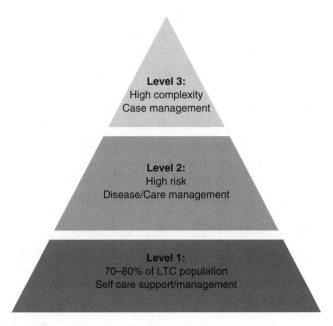

Figure 11.2   The Kaiser permanente pyramid of care

Source: DH (2005b)

services using multidisciplinary teams and disease-specific protocols and pathways, such as the National Service Frameworks (DH, 2005a).

- Level 1: Supported self-care – helping individuals and their carers to develop the knowledge, skills and confidence to care for themselves and their condition effectively (DH, 2005a, 2005b). This builds on an earlier Expert Patient initiative (DH, 2001) which sought to place patients' knowledge of their own conditions at the heart of care.

Central to this system of care is case management, a term used to describe a range of approaches that have been taken to improve the organization and co-ordination of services for people with LTCs. There is no single model of case management, and it exists in many forms in the NHS. However its core elements are: case finding or screening; assessment; care planning; implementation; monitoring and review. These activities can be undertaken by a single 'case manager' or as a series of separate, linked tasks by members of a multidisciplinary team (Hutt et al., 2004). As part of an integrated care model the purpose of case management is to ensure the delivery of co-ordinated care to meet the varied and differing needs of individual clients with LTCs. This service development was also informed by the Evercare model which was piloted in nine PCTs in April 2003 and case management subsequently became part of Government policy for supporting people with LTCs (Busse et al., 2010). Evercare is a model of care for frail older people, developed in the United States by a for-profit health insurance company, which incorporates nurse-led assessment and intensive case management.

Assessing the impact of this aspect of policy is difficult because there is no clear evidence to demonstrate that case management prevents admissions to acute care or reduces the use of emergency services (Hutt et al., 2004; Singh, 2005). This suggests that policy transfer (Hulme, 2005), applying policy pre-scriptions from one health system to another, is not always successful. Similarly an evaluation of the Evercare model pilot in England found that emergency admissions of people with LTCs were unlikely to be reduced by more than 1%, and if greater reductions were to be achieved it would require the appointment of between 20 and 24 Advanced Nurse Practitioners in each PCT (Boaden et al., 2005). With regard to the case manager role, which has been assigned to Community Matrons in the main, there was a commitment to appoint 3,000 by March 2007 to 'spearhead the case management drive' (DH, 2005b). Yet in 2006/7 58% of PCTs had not achieved their target to appoint the planned number of community matrons, and only 32% of 'very high-intensity users' were under their care (Boaden, 2008). Although they are popular with patients and improve the situation for individuals, the case management element of the policy is unlikely to reduce hospital admissions in the absence of a more radical system redesign (Boaden et al., 2006). This emphasizes the point that many health systems are still largely built around an acute, episodic model of care and changing the system to better meet the needs of people with complex LTCs is difficult. The health systems in different countries vary widely and each needs a solution that fits with its overall structure and system model (Nolte et al., 2008). The broad policy commitment is clear, in that everyone with one or more LTC(s) should be offered a personalized care plan, developed, agreed and regularly reviewed with a named lead professional to help manage their care (DH, 2008) with this process managed as part of the system. However if this is to be achieved better co-operation among health and social care organizations needs to be addressed as a priority if deep rooted vested interests and profes-sional scepticism are to be overcome (Busse et al., 2010). This requires good management and political support. A third strand of policy that needs to be adapted to specific national concerns operates at the micro level.

The individual focus: Personalized care planning

The Department of Health has issued guidance on how to incorporate self-care into the policy framework for LTCs (DH, 2009a, 2009b). Effective self-care involves providing appropriate information for individuals and their families, developing a supported process to enable people with LTCs to appraise their current lifestyle choices, think about their individual goals, and build the confidence to attain them. A number of health and social care professionals will be involved in this process, depending on the complexity of the individual's needs (DH, 2009a). Commissioners will require evidence from service providers that the services they 'buy':

- put the individual, their needs, choices, health and well-being at the centre of the process;
- focus on goal setting and clear outcomes;
- are planned, anticipatory and include contingency planning to manage crisis episodes better;
- ensure that people receive co-ordinated care packages, which reduce fragmentation between services;
- provide relevant, timely and accredited information to support client decision making;
- provide support so that people can self-care/self-manage their condition(s) and prevent deterioration;
- promote joined-up working between different professions and agencies, especially between health and social care. (DH, 2009b)

This should result in the collation of all the information about the individual into a single comprehensive paper or electronic care plan, which should also be accessible by the client and those who have a legitimate reason to use it, including out of hours and emergency/urgent care services (DH, 2009b). This micro level policy is designed to give individual patients more leverage in the system. If they learn more about their LTC(s) and the services they can access, it is anticipated that the role of clients as active service users will be enhanced and passive acceptance reduced. It is part of the system-wide policy whereby they become a driver for change as part of the 'demand side' dynamic. However a survey conducted on behalf of the Department of Health (Carluccio et al., 2009) presents a mixed picture of progress in the development of personalized self-care. Information was found to be central in helping people take a greater role in the treatment of their long-term condition with one in five reporting this to be the case. Yet nearly two thirds of the respondents (64%) were not aware of any available training courses that taught self-care skills, and only 4% had accessed a training course of this kind. Although people were generally satisfied with the information and support they received, two in five adults with a LTC had not approached any individual or organization for advice on self-care or information about their LTC (Carluccio et al., 2009). This suggests there is still some way to go before clients are fully engaged in directing their own care.

Recent additions to the policy mix, which have been described as two of the most exciting initiatives to date (Glasby and Duffy, 2007), may

accelerate this process as part of the personalization agenda. Direct payments are cash payments made to disabled people between the ages of
18–65 years in lieu of directly provided services. The payment can then be
used by the individual to purchase services from a voluntary or private
agency (Glasby and Duffy, 2007). This is taken a stage further in the form
of individual budgets which indicate how much individuals have to spend
on their care, and ensure they have control over this funding (Glasby,
2008a). This has the potential to transform the relationship between the
individual and the state from the traditional 'professional gift model',
where the state uses the money it receives from taxation to provide services for clients, to a 'citizenship model', in which the individual is at the
centre of the process and controls the resources to organize the care she/
he wants (Glasby, 2008b). Individual budgets have been tested with 6,000
people since 2003 and have resulted in improvements in personal well-
being and system efficiency (Glasby, 2008a) and these positive results could
offer a framework for reforming the funding of long-term care more generally (Glasby, 2008a). The ultimate outcome of this would be that if providers are to introduce genuine personalization of services they would
need to appeal to 'micro commissioners' (Dickinson and Glasby, 2009),
individuals. This would constitute a significant change in the organization
and delivery of health care, yet it is difficult to predict how policy for LTCs
will develop in England because there is now a new government in office.

Next steps

The policy approach to the provision of care for people with LTC is to be
reviewed. The Conservative and Liberal Democrat Coalition which came
to power in May 2010 published a White Paper which included a number
of proposals that will have a direct impact on policy in this area. One of
the major changes outlined in the White Paper was in the commissioning
process. The government plans to devolve power and responsibility for
commissioning to consortia of General Practitioners (GPs) and their practice teams (DH, 2010b), which will result in PCTs being phased out by
2013. The intention is that by shifting responsibility for commissioning
and budgets to groups of GP practices, services will be shaped around the
needs and choices of patients and that following the passage of the Health
Bill, the consortia will take on full responsibility for commissioning in
2012/13 (DH, 2010b). At the time of writing the precise details of how
this new approach will work are yet to appear, for example: How many
patients will each consortium be responsible for? How many GPs will be
involved in each consortium? What will the management structure be?

And perhaps most importantly what governance arrangements will be put in place? Previous attempts to involve GPs more directly in managing budgets and commissioning services have produced mixed results (Curry et al., 2008; Glennerster et al., 1994; Smith, 2010) and so this new approach to commissioning will need to be managed carefully if it is to be successful.

Although 'choice in care for long-term conditions' as part of personalized care planning is to be available from 2011 (DH 2010b) the extent to which a focus will be maintained on the needs of people with LTCs is not entirely clear and could potentially become less of a priority if the consortia concentrate on commissioning services from secondary care (hospitals). Another significant change that is likely to have far reaching effects on the organization of care for people with LTCs is the establishment of a commission on the funding of long-term care and support which will report in July 2011 (DH, 2010b). The current financial strictures affecting health systems across the world (Newbold and Hyrkäs, 2010) are likely to result in reductions in services as governments seek to correct deficits. For example, the NHS in England will be required to save £15–20 billion in 2011–2014 (Ham, 2009). The review of funding of long-term care will, in all likelihood, lead to different arrangements and the imposition of financial limits and the rationalization of services. However the full picture will not be clear until the commission reports its findings and recommendations. This underlines the need to continually examine the policy context in England and elsewhere, if the organization and delivery of services for people with LTCs are to be understood.

Conclusion

Although there is a comprehensive range of models and guidance to indicate how services for people with LTCs should be organized this can in itself complicate matters further. For example in a document about commissioning personalized care for people with LTCs (DH, 2009b), direction is given to 28 other documents that must be consulted if the process is to be fully understood. When this is considered in the context of a new administration seeking to introduce fundamental reforms it becomes clear that although policy statements may emphasize the need to focus on clients and ensure high quality service delivery, these aspirations can be sidelined in the efforts to overhaul the system and make savings. In common with many other areas of health policy the management arrangements for people with LTCs are subject to frequent change. Reviewing policy using a model such as the one outlined here is necessary to track the origins and implications of such changes.

Summary

This chapter has shown how the macro, meso, micro approach to policy analysis can provide a useful framework for examining the organization of care for people with long-term conditions in England. It is clear that there is no single policy model for the management of the health and social care for people with long-term conditions and policy approaches have to be adapted to the context of different systems. The role of the new GP Commissioning Consortia in England will be crucial to service delivery in this area.

Note

1 Beacon sites are usually individual departments that are using innovative approaches to address problems or promote best practice in health and social care. The NHS Beacon programme was launched with 290 sites in 1999.

Further reading

Jones, K. and Netten, A. (2010) 'The costs of change: A case study of the process of implementing individual budgets across pilot local authorities in England', *Health & Social Care in the Community*, 18(10): 51–8.

Naylor, C. and Goodwin, N. (2010) *Building High Quality Commissioning – What Role Can External Organisations Play?* London: King's Fund.

References

Barrett, S. and Fudge, C. (1981) 'Examining the policy-action relationship', in S. Barrett and C. Fudge (eds), *Policy and Action: Essays on the Implementation of Public Policy*. London: Methuen. pp. 3–32.

Bergen, A. and While, A. (2005) 'Implementation deficit and street-level bureaucracy: Policy, practice and change in the development of community nursing issues', *Health and Social Care in the Community*, 13(1): 1–10.

Boaden, R. (2008) 'Can community matrons cut hospital admissions?', *Pulse*, 27 March [Online]. Available at: http://www.pulsetoday.co.uk/story.asp?storycode= 4118121 (accessed 4 August 2010).

Boaden, R., Dusheiko, M., Gravelle, H., Parker, S., Pickard, S., Roland, M., Sheaff, R. and Sargent, P. (2005) *Evercare Evaluation Interim Report: Implications for Supporting People with Long-term Conditions*. Manchester: National Primary Care Research Centre, University of Manchester.

Boaden, R., Dusheiko, M., Gravelle, H., Parker, S., Pickard, S., Roland, M., Sargent, P. and Sheaff, R. (2006) *Evercare Evaluation: Final Report*. Manchester: National Primary Care Research and Development Centre.

Busse, R., Blümel, M., Scheller-Kreinsen, D. and Zentner, A. (2010) *Tackling Chronic Disease in Europe: Strategies, Interventions and Challenges*. Denmark: World Health Organization, on behalf of the European Observatory on Health Systems and Policies.

Canadian Health Services Research Foundation (2005) 'Interdisciplinary teams in primary health care can effectively manage chronic illness', *Evidence Boost*, September, [Online] Available at: www.chsrfa.ca, 1-2 (accessed May 2006).

Carluccio, A., Carroll, P. and Worley, T. (2009) *Long-term Health Conditions 2009*. Research Study Conducted for the Department of Health. London: IpsosMORI/DH.

Chote, R. (2007) 'Health and the public spending squeeze. Funding prospects for the NHS', in J. Appleby (ed.), *Funding Health Care 2008 and Beyond. Report from the Leeds Castle Summit* . London: King's Fund. pp. 35–42.

Crinson, I. (2009) *Health Policy – A Critical Perspective*. London: Sage.

Curry, N., Godwin, N., Naylor, C. and Robertson, R. (2008) *Practice-based Commissioning: Replace, Reinvigorate or Abandon?* London: King's Fund.

De Silva, D. and Fahey, D. (2008) 'England', in E. Nolte, C. Knai and M. McKee (eds), *Managing Chronic Conditions Experience in Eight Countries*. World Health Organization, on behalf of the European Observatory on Health Systems and Policies. Denmark: WHO.

DH (2001) *The Expert Patient: A New Approach to Chronic Disease Management for the 21st century*. London: Department of Health.

DH (2004) *Annual Report*. London: The Stationery Office.

DH (2005a) *The National Service Framework for Long-Term Conditions*. London: Department of Health.

DH (2005b) *Supporting People with Long-term Conditions* (4230). London: Department of Health.

DH (2008) *High Quality Care for All NHS Next Stage Review-Final Report*. London: Department of Health.

DH (2009a) *Your Health, Your Way. A Guide to Long-term Conditions and Self Care*. London: Department of Health.

DH (2009b) *Supporting People with Long-term Conditions – Commissioning Personalised Care Planning*. London: Department of Health.

DH (2010a) *Improving the Health and Well-being of People with Long-term Conditions: World Class Services for People with Long-term Conditions – Information Tool for Commissioners*. London: Department of Health.

DH (2010b) *Equity and Excellence: Liberating the NHS*. London: Department of Health.

Dickinson, H. and Glasby, J (2009) *The Personalisation Agenda: Implications for the Third Sector*. Briefing paper 30. Birmingham: Third Sector Research Centre.

Dixon, J. (2007) 'Improving management of chronic illness in the National Health Service: Better incentives are the key', *Chronic Illness*, 3: 181–93.

Dorey, P. (2005) *Policy Making in Britain: An Introduction*. London: Sage Publications.

Dunn, W. N. (2004) *Public Policy Analysis – An Introduction*, 3rd edn. New Jersey: Pearson/Prentice Hall.

Earle, S. (2007) 'Promoting public health in a global context', in C.E. Lloyd, S. Handsley, J. Douglas, S. Earle and S. Spurr (eds), *Policy and Practice in Promoting Public Health*. London: Sage Publications. pp. 1–32.

Glasby, J. (2008a) *Individual Patient Budgets: Background and Frequently Asked Questions*. HSMC Policy Paper 1. Birmingham: Health Services Management Centre, University of Birmingham.

Glasby, J. (2008b) 'Who Cares?' Policy Proposals for the Reform of Long-Term Care. Birmingham: Health Services Management Centre, University of Birmingham.

Glasby, J. and Duffy, S. (2007) Our Health, Our Care, Our Say – What Could the NHS Learn from Individual Budgets and Direct Payments? Joint HSMC and in Control discussion paper. Birmingham: Health Services Management Centre, University of Birmingham.

Glennerster, H., Matsaganis, M., Owens, P. and Hancock, S. (1994) Implementing GP Fundholding: Wild Card or Winning Hand? Buckingham: Open University Press.

Ham, C. (2005) 'Lost in translation? Health systems in the US and the UK', Social Policy and Administration, 39(2): 192–209.

Ham, C. (2009) Health in a Cold Climate – Developing an Intelligent Response to Financial Challenges Facing the NHS. Briefing Paper. London: The Nuffield Trust.

Ham, C. (2010) Working Together for Health: Achievements and Challenges in the Kaiser NHS Beacon Sites Programme. Birmingham: Health Services Management Centre, University of Birmingham.

Ham, C. and Hill, M. (1993) The Policy Process in the Modern Capitalist State. New York: Harvester Wheatsheaf.

Hudson, J. and Lowe, S. (2004) Understanding the Policy Process. Bristol: The Policy Press.

Hulme, R. (2005) 'Policy transfer and the internationalisation of social policy', Social Policy & Society, 4(4): 417–25.

Hunter, D.J. (2003) Public Health Policy. Cambridge: Polity.

Hutt, R., Rosen, R. and McCauley, J. (2004) Case-Managing Long-Term Conditions: What Impact does it have in the Treatment of Older People? London: King's Fund.

Lindblom, C E. (1959) 'The science of 'muddling through', Public Administration Review, 19: 78–88.

Lindblom, C. E. (1979) 'Still muddling, not yet through', Public Administration Review, 39: 517–25.

Newbold, D. and Hyrkäs, K. (2010) 'Managing in economic austerity', Journal of Nursing Management, 18(5): 495–500.

Nolte, E., McKee, M. and Knai, C. (2008) 'Managing chronic conditions: An introduction to the experience in eight countries', in E. Nolte, C. Knai and M. McKedd (eds), Managing Chronic Conditions – Experience in Eight Countries. World Health Organization, on behalf of the European Observatory on Health Systems and Policies. Denmark: WHO. pp. 1–14.

Prime Minister's Strategy Unit (2006) The UK Government's Approach to Public Service Reform [Online]. Available at: www.cabinetoffice.gov.uk/media/cabinetoffice/strategy/assess/sj_pamphlet.pdf (accessed 3 November 2008).

Singh, D. (2005) Transforming Chronic Care: Evidence about Improving Care of People with Long-term Conditions. Birmingham: Health Services Management Centre, University of Birmingham.

Singh, D. (2008) How Can Chronic Disease Management Programmes Operate Across Care Settings? Copenhagen: World Health Organization Europe.

Smith, J. (2010) Giving GPs Budgets for Commissioning: What Needs to be Done? London: The Nuffield Trust.

World Health Organization (2005) Preventing Chronic Disease: A Vital Investment. WHO Global Report. Geneva: WHO.

World Health Organization (n.d.) Solving the Chronic Disease Problem. www.who.int/chp/chronic_disease_report/media/Factsheet5.pdf (accessed 20 October 2010).

12

International Experience of Integrating Health and Social Care for People Living with HIV

Erica Richardson

Overview

- How did HIV become a long-term condition?
- The diverse care needs of people living with HIV
- Integration in practice – HIV care for asylum seekers
- Holistic care: Person-centred or patient-centred?
- Historical context for integrating health and social care for people living with HIV
- The continuing importance of grassroots community groups

In the European Union in 2009 there were 343,093 people known to be living with HIV (ECDC and WHO Europe, 2010). HIV is a virus which weakens the body's immune system thus making people living with the virus more susceptible to diseases. HIV can be transmitted through unprotected sexual intercourse with someone living with HIV, sharing infected injecting equipment, and 'vertically' from a mother living with HIV to her child during pregnancy, childbirth or breastfeeding; HIV is not transmitted through everyday contact. In Western Europe new

HIV diagnoses have been increasing, and so too is the total number of people living with HIV, but the latter is largely due to the wide access to treatment which keeps the virus under control and supports the immune system and prevents the progression to AIDS. In countries of Western Europe where there is broad access to health care, people living with HIV are able to access effective drug treatments and living with HIV has been reframed as a long-term condition (LTC) by health and social care organizations. In this respect, HIV is a relatively 'new' LTC, which is markedly different to LTCs which are non-communicable diseases. The nature of transmission routes means that HIV infection is highly stigmatized and the communities in all EU countries which have been most seriously affected by the disease (for example injecting drug users) are also marginalized. Part of the stigmatization of living with HIV is also the popular misconception that it is an inevitable 'death sentence' (Richardson, 2009).

The nature of the condition, the nature of the treatment regime, and the nature of the groups most heavily affected mean that HIV is a particularly illuminating example to use when exploring the integration of health and social care. The integration of health and social care for people living with HIV is different to other long-term conditions as it evolved within grass-roots community groups and was then co-opted by state providers rather than being a state-led initiative. The aim of this chapter is to provide a greater understanding of the complexity of integrating care by exploring the boundaries and policy drivers for HIV services in high-income countries. First, the nature of HIV as a long-term condition and its treatment regimes are outlined to highlight the particular complexity of needs in health and social care integration. Secondly, the historical response to the challenges of integrating care for people living with HIV is described to explore the basis for integrated health and social care services. The chapter then concludes with a review of the key messages for practitioners, researchers and policy makers.

HIV as a long-term condition (LTC)

There are some transient physical symptoms associated with initial HIV infection, such as flu-like symptoms and diarrhoea. However, unless HIV remains untreated and the infection progresses so that the individual is seriously immuno-compromised or can be said to have developed AIDS (if a particular range of conditions are present), it may not be the HIV infection itself which causes the physical difficulties, but the treatment.

There are possible side-effects of antiretrovirals which mean that people living with HIV may have to cope with chronic pain, changes to their physical appearance, endocrinological problems, as well as a complex drug regimen and the possible interactions with different foods. Initially it was felt that people with HIV would be willing to live with the side-effects and the restrictions on lifestyle that taking antiretroviral drugs entailed because it gave them a longer life, but this is not always so (Gazzard and Jones, 2006). If a person with HIV does not access treatment, for example, because they are unaware of their positive status, they are likely to remain asymptomatic until their immune system is seriously compromised. Once this occurs, they are vulnerable to a range of diseases with which their immune system could normally cope; at this point they are likely to be considered to have developed AIDS. Before the development of effective treatments, most people with HIV died of AIDS-related illnesses.

The development of antiretrovirals has had a dramatic impact on HIV-related mortality and morbidity which have enabled HIV infection to shift from being a terminal to a chronic disease. However, antiretrovirals are still a treatment and not a cure. HIV is a lifelong condition which requires constant medication under close medical supervision. Effective antiretroviral agents have been available for the treatment of HIV since 1987, although early treatments were unsustainable or were only partially effective (Lange, 2006). From 1996 more effective multi-drug therapies have been available and, currently, the most effective treatment for HIV is highly active antiretroviral therapy (HAART). This combined drug regime slows down replication of the virus and helps prevent the virus from becoming resistant to drugs so the treatment remains effective.

The main medical challenges of antiretroviral therapy are those of adherence and toxicity. The drug combination is a delicate balancing act and 95% adherence to treatment is required to avoid HIV developing drug resistance, which would limit future treatment options for the individual (Lange, 2006). Adherence can be difficult because different pills often need to be taken at different specific times throughout the day, every day, either with or without food. Adherence to drug regimes varies depending on the type of drug being prescribed, the length of time for which it should be taken and the complexity of the drug regimen, which is tailored to the individual. Adherence thus depends on the social context in which illness and treatment are experienced rather than on the characteristics of individual patients. For this reason, the term 'adherence' is resisted by many people living with long-term conditions as it has connotations of being a 'good' or 'bad' patient who is subordinate to a powerful all-knowing clinician, rather than an equal partner in the management of a particular condition. Therefore, even though the term 'adherence' is still used in relation to HIV care, it is the social context in which it can be achieved that is of key importance in understanding the social as well as health needs of people living with HIV. While most people on HIV treatment can live active and healthy lives, others experience side-effects from the drugs due to their toxicity. The toxicity of antiretrovirals relates to a number of disfiguring, debilitating and potentially fatal side effects which have been reduced as new regimens have been developed, but often insufficient attention is paid to the side-effects of treatment and the long-term mental health impact of living with HIV in health and social care settings (Harding and Molloy, 2008).

The mental health impact of living with HIV is strongly associated with the level of stigma surrounding the virus and how stigmatized people living with HIV can be made to feel. Societal attitudes towards HIV and people living with HIV are disabling and they can face discrimination and harassment if their positive status becomes common knowledge. Although it is not specifically named in EU anti-discrimination legislation, HIV positive status is now recognized as a disability by many governments in Europe, often from the point of diagnosis whether or not the individual has accessed treatment. HIV is 'disabling' in view of the side-effects of the treatment regime, the unpredictability of the ways in which the needs of people living with HIV change and the mental health impact of living with a stigmatized condition.

Integrated care models have been developed mainly in relation to the complex needs of older people with multiple long-term conditions whereas people living with HIV (PLHIV) are often much younger and face a different range of co-morbidities such as other chronic infections (e.g. hepatitis C) or opportunistic infections to which PLHIV are more vulnerable due to their immuno-compromised status (e.g. tuberculosis). However, the complex health and social care needs of people living with HIV have been shaped most strongly by the epidemiology of the infection, which has disproportionately affected certain marginalized communities such as men who have sex with men (MSM), injecting drug users (IDUs), sex workers and some migrant populations. Also, people living with HIV do not fit neatly into just one group – indeed, potentially they could encompass all four (i.e. be a migrant IDU MSM who sells sex) or none of the above. The diversity of people living with HIV presents many challenges to the integration of health and social care which have been addressed in different ways depending on the local context and in response to the local populations most at risk. MSM continue to be the population group most at risk of exposure to HIV within most Western European countries (ECDC and WHO Europe, 2010). However, the use of contaminated injecting equipment among drug users remains the main mode of transmission in Estonia, Latvia, Lithuania and Poland, despite it accounting for a decreasing proportion of new cases in Western Europe (ECDC and WHO Europe, 2010).

The age range of people living with HIV, and its relatively recent shift to becoming a long-term condition, means that some of their social care needs encompass education and employment programmes. People living with HIV need support in their work environment but also in returning to the workplace, particularly as many face discrimination if their diagnosis becomes common knowledge (Harding and Molloy, 2008). For many people living with HIV, their positive status has no impact on their working lives, although those who experience side-effects from some treatment regimes are more likely to require their health needs to be taken into account by employers. For example, peripheral neuropathy can limit an individual's ability to walk long distances or stand for long periods. Housing can also be an acute need for people living with HIV (Cameron et al., 2007). In the UK, research has shown that one in three people living with HIV have experienced poverty, leaving them vulnerable to housing problems and homelessness (NAT, 2010). Poverty and homelessness can also be some of the most pressing needs for people living with HIV who have insecure immigration status or who are seeking asylum (Allan and Clarke, 2005). For some people with HIV, living in vulnerable housing can be the result of domestic violence (Ciambrone, 2001). In addition to such potential social care needs, people living with HIV also benefit from access to integrated mental health and addictions services (Harding and Molloy, 2008; Hoang et al., 2009; Lemmon and Shuff, 2001), sexual and reproductive health services (Church and Lewin, 2010), as well as services related to any co-infections such as hepatitis or tuberculosis (Hoang et al., 2009). However, one of the most basic needs for HIV positive persons on diagnosis is information – about their condition, about treatment options, about their legal position and about any access they may have to benefits and services (Allan and Clarke, 2005). In order to help illustrate these points, a case study based on an evaluation by Allan and Clarke (2005) has been included below.

Case Study Integration in practice: Addressing the health and social care needs of HIV positive asylum seekers (after Allan and Clarke, 2005)

Allan and Clarke (2005) conducted an evaluation of HIV and sexual health services for HIV-positive persons with insecure immigration or asylum seekers in Leeds. They mapped current service provision and identified any unmet needs. In the UK, asylum seekers do not have access to the full range of benefits and social care services which are available to formal UK residents.

The Centre for Sexual Health, based in the Genito-Urinary Medicine Clinic of a large hospital, is the health care provider responsible for treating the HIV positive clients. All those diagnosed as HIV positive are offered support and counselling by Health Advisors, who can also link people living with HIV into other service providers. For example, asylum seekers and people with insecure immigration status can be referred to the Health Access Team, also a statutory health provider, which can support them in accessing mainstream health services.

The Terrence Higgins Trust (THT), one of the leading national HIV and AIDS charities in the UK, was named as an important source of information and advice on living well with HIV – particularly with regard to coping with side-effects of treatment. As well as addressing these health needs, THT also assisted clients in addressing social needs such as finding suitable housing.

The largest national children's charity, Barnardo's, also ran a confidential service run by African workers for African families and individuals living with HIV providing peer support and some hardship funds. While the service was made more accessible in being run by Africans for Africans, it was also a barrier as some clients worried about confidentiality and would not use the service in case they met someone they knew.

The description of services provided in the assessment shows that health and social care integration is happening and that the care provided is 'person-centred' (see below). However, this is largely happening outside the state health providers which conduct the diagnosis and treatment of HIV and help asylum seekers to navigate the health system. It also happens on an *ad hoc* basis and relies on the Health Advisors in the Centre for Sexual Health being aware of the broader difficulties faced by asylum seekers; housing or immigration status may actually be more important in the client's life than their HIV positive status.

Patient-centred or person-centred care?

Before effective treatments became available, HIV care services were rooted in communicable disease control, sexual health and palliative care services. With the shift to HIV management as a long-term condition, the need for greater integration of services and more holistic care has become more pressing. Holistic care is where the client is viewed as a whole person, with individual preferences situated within a social-environmental context (Church and

Lewin, 2010). However, the focus of most research into the integration of services for people living with HIV has focused more on the complexity of their health care needs with regard to co-morbidities rather than the need to address both social and health care needs in conjunction. The health care needs are thus the focus of attention rather than the individual. Integration of health and social care services is necessary for improved compliance with HAART regimes and so-called 'virtuous circles of care' which result in less drug resistance and a lower viral load (Hoang et al., 2009). This is particularly important as the successful treatment of HIV might not be the most pressing care need from the perspective of the individual client for whom other issues such as poverty, homelessness, domestic violence or insecure immigration status could actually be more significant (Allan and Clarke, 2005; Ciambrone, 2001; Kennedy and Rogers, 2009).

There is a fundamental tension in the integration of services which reflects competing discourses, one rooted in a health care perspective, which focuses on 'patient-centred care', and one rooted in a social care perspective, which focuses on 'person-centred care' (Nolte and McKee, 2008). The 'person' versus 'patient' divide reflects differing approaches to the role of the person/patient in the management of their condition. The health care perspective comes from a biomedical discourse which views the patient as a more or less passive consumer of health care services rather than as a proactive partner in decision-making on treatment options. By contrast, the person-centred discourses often seek to 'demedicalize' care by underlining the interdependencies between health and social care in meeting the needs of individual service users (Nolte and McKee, 2008). The boundaries between these discourses are negotiated differently from one country to another and broadly reflect the way in which health and social care services are financed and organized in a given country, but services for people living with HIV have also been shaped by the nature of the condition and the epidemic.

There have been numerous attempts to create a taxonomy of models of integration for people living with long-term conditions in order to develop an 'evidence base' for policy makers by assessing the structures and processes involved, their prerequisites and their effect on service organization and delivery, and user outcomes (Nolte and McKee, 2008). For people living with HIV, research is conducted predominantly from a health care perspective so is quite narrowly focused on the integration of different branches of the health system and treatment outcomes. However, in practice HIV care in high-income countries does often involve the integration of health and social services even though this is rarely discussed in the research literature.

Integrating health and social care for people living with HIV

Models for the development of health and social care initiatives have emphasized the importance of community involvement at all stages of the process, and usually policy makers have sought to achieve this through the involvement of grassroots community groups and non-government organizations. This inevitably involves shifts in power relationships and resources from dominant state organizations (usually in health care) to build community capacity. However, this is not the pattern which has been followed in the development of HIV and AIDS services in high-income countries where community groups have consistently had a stronger role as service providers and co-ordinators. The strong involvement of the voluntary sector is a legacy of early responses to the HIV and AIDS epidemic in the 1980s. Early government and societal inaction was rooted in the stigmatization of the virus itself and the marginalized groups which were predominantly affected at that time. In Western Europe and North America the movement for lesbian, gay, bisexual and transgender (LGBT) rights has been at the vanguard of advocacy efforts for the treatment and prevention of HIV and AIDS, largely because MSM were the first group to be seriously affected. The 'AIDS Movement', as it was known initially, inherited much of its political activism from the LGBT movement, but the groups most at risk varies from country to country, and some groups such as IDUs were less politically active.

IDUs (the first group to be seriously affected by HIV in Southern Europe) often lacked the grassroots community group infrastructure with which to advocate change. The Junkie Union in The Netherlands is a notable exception in that they were already very active in developing services to support the health needs of IDUs – they founded the first needle exchange programme in 1984 in response to an outbreak of hepatitis B. The significance of community groups in service provision is well demonstrated in the case of 'harm reduction' initiatives for IDUs such as syringe and needle exchanges, methadone maintenance programmes and education programmes promoting safer injecting practices. In many countries such programmes were politically untenable and as such it was not possible for such services to be directly funded and provided by the state. Instead, grassroots community organizations were at the forefront of HIV services for IDUs, as they had the freedom to embrace the harm reduction approach and, importantly, they had access to, and the trust of IDUs. Many harm reduction initiatives have subsequently been co-opted by state providers; elsewhere (where harm reduction is still politically divisive) community organizations have remained core service providers (Lane et al., 2000).

The mobilization of people living with HIV themselves happened early in the epidemic and they have consequently become key stakeholders. People living with HIV have also been central to moving HIV up the policy agenda as well as ensuring that as the client group they are central to the health and social care services which target them, whether the funding is from state or charitable sources. The AIDS Movement quickly became global; lobbying transnational organizations for greater recognition and more resources, which resulted in the founding of global organizations such as UNAIDS (Guarinieri and Hollander, 2006). However, the response to HIV and AIDS was never fully relinquished to state health or social care organizations and due to the continued stigmatization of HIV and discrimination against PLHIV the advocacy role of community groups has continued; in part because state sector providers cannot necessarily be 'trusted' to provide adequate care (Park, 2006).

The importance of grassroots community groups

The extensive role of community groups in pushing forward care of PLHIV means that their involvement is now considered essential for the provision of high quality services. In countries where there has been weak community participation in HIV services there have been poor health outcomes (Guarinieri and Hollander, 2006). For example, the limited involvement of HIV and AIDS community groups in service provision in Central and East European countries has been highlighted as one reason for the lack of success in controlling the HIV epidemic in that region (Atun, 2006). Working with community groups provides much better scope for co-ordinating health and social care by ensuring they are responsive to the disparate needs of different client groups. Community groups appear less constrained by organizational priorities and professional agenda and more able to respond flexibly to meet the complex needs of individuals in HIV services (Cameron et al., 2007). Consequently, there is a strong ethos of encouraging multiagency working although it has also been noted that groups representing the different interests and needs of people living with HIV have not necessarily worked well together (Guarinieri and Hollander, 2006). Community organizations can also be of critical importance in allowing access to particularly hard-to-reach groups who can be highly marginalized and reluctant to access services provided through the statutory system. For example, clients with insecure immigration status may avoid making services aware of their presence in the country and the same can be true for clients involved in criminalized behaviours such as sex work or drug use.

The strong involvement of community groups in the co-ordination of health and social care services for people living with HIV has had a positive impact on health outcomes for the client group and has greatly facilitated the integration of health and social care services where it has occurred. However, community groups by their very nature have precarious funding and depending on the way in which state-funded services are organized and the way in which community groups are involved in service provision and co-ordination, can mean that integrated services are extremely vulnerable to budget cuts. In trying to control spending, some state providers can try to 'offload' the cost of such services to other sectors (e.g. from the health system to the social care system or the voluntary sector). This is significant because 'patient-centred' services which are funded from treatment and care budgets can be viewed as secondary to HIV social care, support and information services (Weatherburn et al., 2007).

Integration works best where the services are determined by the characteristics of those who use it rather than pre-existing organizational structures, and often agencies outside statutory structures are best placed to enable this (Cameron et al., 2007). Research on integrating services for people living with HIV has also shown that the more longstanding collaboration between statutory agencies and community groups has been, the more likely it will be to lead to a fruitful partnership based on mutual understanding and trust (Cameron et al., 2007). The successful integration of care also relies on the successful integration of information systems between agencies and this can be one of the core barriers to multidisciplinary working. There can be legislative barriers to health care providers sharing information with social providers (and vice versa) and the need to protect a client's confidentiality can also hinder information sharing between statutory and community organizations. This is of particular importance for people living with HIV where stigma means that confidentiality is very often a core concern for service users.

So what works?

The stigmatization of HIV and subsequent challenges in accessing services tests the boundaries of health and social care integration. People living with HIV as a long-term condition have many complex needs which cannot be met in the health or social care sectors acting in isolation – the maintenance of health and functional capacity requires more types of service than any one part of a system can deliver alone (Lemmon and Shuff, 2001). The history and epidemiology of HIV has meant that integration in high-income countries has most effectively been achieved by or mediated through the involvement of grassroots community groups. It has been argued that the strengths and successes of this approach is something which could be useful for the integration of services for other long-term conditions (Cameron et al., 2007). The broadening of access to HAART also means that health and social care systems in low- and middle-income countries are facing a growing need for integrated service provision not only across clinical disciplines, but also between health and social care providers through the development of more client-centred services (Church and Lewin, 2010). However, it is not clear how achievable this may be in the medium term.

Research has also shown that often successful integration of health and social care services is founded on good personal relations between key stakeholders involved where trust and mutual respect has developed over long-term collaborations (Cameron et al., 2007; Lemmon and Shuff, 2001). This is not something which can necessarily be implemented 'top-down' as a policy measure, although awareness of the issue can foster the development of such relations by ensuring that all stakeholders across the sectors are brought on-board from the design stage in any integrating projects (Cameron et al., 2007). The importance of long-term collaborations between partners could also be reflected in the way integrated services are funded (Weatherburn et al., 2007). Similarly, the central role of grassroots community groups in the successful provision of integrated health and social care services is not something that can be easily 'borrowed' by countries which do not have a strong recent history of community participation (Atun, 2006). Such contextual differences between living with HIV relative to other long-term conditions, or national constraints around the way health and social care services are organized, or the capacity of grassroots community groups to take on service provision or co-ordination, are significant and highlight the difficulties and pitfalls in transnational comparisons and transnational learning. Understanding the context is therefore of crucial importance, but the challenges are not insurmountable and can help to illustrate the inherent tensions in what integration means in practice.

Summary

HIV has been reframed as a long-term condition since the development of effective treatment regimes. These treatment regimes can have debilitating side-effects, but without treatment most people living with HIV will develop AIDS. People living with HIV have diverse care needs which reflect the nature of the condition and its treatment but also the marginalized groups which have been disproportionately affected by HIV. Unlike other long-term conditions, grassroots community groups in the voluntary sector have been at the forefront of integrated health and social care service provision in HIV care. There are benefits and challenges in the extensive role played by the voluntary sector in service provision, but overall international experience shows that it is the most effective way of meeting the diverse care needs of people living with HIV.

Further reading

Beck, E.J., Mays, N., Whiteside, A.W. and Zuniga, J.M. (eds) (2006) *The HIV Pandemic: Local and Global Implications.* New York: Oxford University Press.

Matic, S., Lazarus, J.V. and Donoghoe, M.C. (eds) (2006) *HIV/AIDS in Europe: Moving from Death Sentence to Chronic Disease Management.* Copenhagen: WHO Regional Office for Europe.

References

Allan, C. L. and Clarke, J. (2005) 'Are HIV/AIDS services in Leeds, UK, able to meet the needs of asylum seekers?', *Public Health*, 119(4): 305–11.

Atun, R.A. (2006) 'How European health systems have reacted to the HIV/AIDS epidemic', in S. Matic, J.V. Lazarus and M.C. Donoghoe (eds), *HIV/AIDS in Europe: Moving from Death Sentence to Chronic Disease Management.* Copenhagen: WHO Regional Office for Europe. pp. 134–54.

Cameron, A., Macdonald, G., Turner, W. and Lloyd, L. (2007) 'The challenges of joint working: Lessons from the Supporting People Health Pilot evaluation', *International Journal of Integrated Care*, 7(1): 1–10.

Church, K. and Lewin, S. (2010) 'Delivering integrated HIV services: Time for a cli-ent-centred approach to meet the sexual and reproductive health needs of people living with HIV?', *AIDS*, 24(2): 189–93.

Ciambrone, D. (2001) 'Illness and other assaults on self: The relative impact of HIV/ AIDS on women's lives', *Sociology of Health and Illness*, 23(4): 517–40.

European Centre for Disease Prevention and Control (ECDC) and WHO Regional Office for Europe (2010) *HIV/AIDS Surveillance in Europe 2009.* Stockholm: ECDC.

Gazzard, B.G. and Jones, R.S. (2006) 'From death to life: Two decades of progress in HIV therapy', in S. Matic, J.V. Lazarus and M.C. Donoghoe (eds), *HIV/AIDS in Europe: Moving from Death Sentence to Chronic Disease Management.* Copenhagen: WHO Regional Office for Europe. pp.101–17.

Guarinieri, M. and Hollander, L. (2006) 'From Denver to Dublin: the role of civil society in HIV treatment and control', in S. Matic, J.V. Lazarus and M.C. Donoghoe (eds), *HIV/AIDS in Europe: Moving from Death Sentence to Chronic Disease Management.* Copenhagen: WHO Regional Office for Europe. pp. 86–100.

Harding, R. and Molloy, T. (2008) 'Positive futures? The impact of HIV infection on achieving health, wealth and future planning', *AIDS Care*, 20(5): 565–70.

Hoang, T., Goetz, M. B., Yano, E., Rossman, B., Anaya, H., Knapp, H., Korthuis, P. T., Henry, R., Bowman, C., Gifford, A. and Asch, S. M. (2009) 'The impact of integrated HIV care on patient health outcomes', *Medical Care*, 47(5): 560–7.

Kennedy, A.P. and Rogers, A.E. (2009) 'The needs of others: The norms of self-management skills training and the differing priorities of asylum seekers with HIV', *Health Sociology Review*, 18(2): 145–58.

Lane, S.D., Lurie, P., Bowser, B., Kahn, J. and Chen, D. (2000) 'The coming of age of needle exchange: A history through 1993', in J.A. Inciardi and L.D. Harrison (eds), *Harm Reduction: National and International Perspectives*. Thousand Oaks, CA: Sage Publications, Inc. pp. 47–68.

Lange, J.M.A. (2006) 'Antiretroviral treatment and care of HIV', in E.J. Beck, N. Mays, A.W. Whiteside and J.M. Zuniga (eds), *The HIV Pandemic: Local and Global Implications.* New York: Oxford University Press. pp. 86–104.

Lemmon, R. and Shuff, I.M. (2001) 'Effects of mental health centre staff turnover on HIV/AIDS service delivery integration', *AIDS Care*. 13(5:) 651–61.

National AIDS Trust (NAT) (2010) *HIV and Housing: A Practical Guide for Housing Officers on HIV and its Impact on Housing Needs.* London: NAT.

Nolte, E. and McKee, M. (2008) 'Integration and chronic care: A review', in E. Nolte and M. McKee (eds), *Caring for People with Chronic Conditions: A Health System Perspective.* Maidenhead: Open University Press. pp. 64–91.

Park, C. (2006) 'Empowering people living with HIV in Europe: Manifesto, mantra or mirage?', in S. Matic, J.V. Lazarus and M.C. Donoghoe (eds), *HIV/AIDS in Europe: Moving from Death Sentence to Chronic Disease Management.* Copenhagen: WHO Regional Office for Europe. pp. 15–26.

Richardson, E. (2009) 'HIV/AIDS: A highly stigmatized long-term condition', in S. Earle and E. Denny (eds), *The Sociology of Long-term Conditions.* Basingstoke and New York: Palgrave Macmillan.

Weatherburn, P., Keough, P., Dodds, C., Hickson, F. and Henderson, L. (2007). *The Growing Challenge: A Strategic Review of HIV Social Care, Support and Information Services across the UK.* London: Sigma Research.

13

Worth a Risk? Risk Taking and People with Long-term Conditions

Tom Heller

Overview

- People with long-term conditions may decide to take risks in relation to the management of their condition
- Health and social care professionals and their employing organizations are more likely to be risk averse
- Risk assessment is something that is done to people with long-term conditions who are expected to remain passive recipients
- 'Risk assessment' is increasingly used in professional practice – but remains an imperfect tool

There is always a power differential between health and social care professionals (especially doctors and social workers), and the people who come to see them seeking help. When people have a long-term condition – particularly longstanding mental distress – this differential becomes even more marked. The professionals often have the power to make significant decisions over the life and even the liberty of the people who are going through a difficult period in their lives. Often the decisions taken by those in authority are dressed up in terms of risk: 'you are at risk of harming yourself' or 'you are at risk of harming those around you'. But the assessment of risk is fraught with problems – it is by no means a perfect science. Health and social care organizations often work towards trying to eliminate all risks for fear of being held responsible for any untoward occurrences – but the people who are 'risk-assessed' might have a different attitude towards risk and how they want to live their lives. For many people taking risks is an important part of their identity ... and this very much includes people with long-term conditions.

Although the total absence of risk is not possible for individuals, for health and social care organizations or for society as a whole, some commentators have noted a general trend towards attempts at risk avoidance in all these spheres (Neuberger, 2008). Health and social care organizations often spend a lot of energy thinking about ways in which risk can be minimized. However this trend may have unintended consequences;

> We are seriously risk averse whenever we offer help or care professionally, and that leads to unkindness as it is easier to do nothing than to run the risk of blame. (Neuberger, 2008: 1)

This chapter aims to consider some of the ways that risk taking and professional risk assessment affects the lives of people with long-term conditions. People with long-term mental health issues in their lives are particularly prone to having formal risk assessments done *to* them – and this situation is used as an example within the chapter.

Individual attitudes to risk

Each individual person develops their own unique attitude to risk – and of course people with long-term conditions do so as well. For each of us a degree of risk-taking is a central part of our personality and an integral part of the way that human beings think and behave. Peoples' attitude to risk is acknowledged as an important descriptor of their individuality and a pointer towards understanding their behaviour.

Annie Dillard, an American author, famously said:

> If we listened to our intellect, we'd never have a love affair. We'd never have a friendship. We'd never go into business, because we'd be too cynical. Well, that's nonsense. You've got to jump off cliffs all the time and build your wings on the way down.

Perhaps taking risks is an integral part of doing creative things, but it may also be a central part of the lives of all of us – including those of us with long-term conditions. Some people remain anxious and 'risk-averse' while others seem positively impelled to seek out risky situations from which to learn their own limits and challenges (Lupton and Tulloch, 2002).

Of course not all risks involve possibly jeopardizing our physical comfort or safety. Speaking out about a subject that is important might involve a particular sort of risk. Trying something new, like singing in a choir, might constitute a risk to your self esteem, but not involve much in the way of physical dangers or personal sacrifice ... and becoming an activist to forward the rights of people with long-term conditions also involves a particular attitude to risk taking.

Risk and personality

The way that individuals assess and deal with risky elements in their lives forms a significant component of their personality (Nicholson et al., 2005; Zuckerman and Kuhlman, 2000). It has been hypothesized (Llewellyn, 2008) that there may be three fundamental approaches to risk: 'risk avoiders', who do all they can to contain the risks they perceive in the world around them, 'risk reducers' who may do risky things on occasion in spite of the risks, and 'risk optimizers' who are positively motivated by exposure to risk. Marvin Zuckerman (2006), an American psychologist, studied people who seemed to be attracted to risk-taking behaviour and attempted to construct their psychological profiles. These risk-taking people were found to be venturesome, inquisitive and eager to have new and exciting experiences ... but do they share a 'sensation seeking trait' and is this genetically determined or the result of their upbringing and the social situation in which they find themselves?

There is a great range of risk-taking behaviours and most people, including those with a long-term condition, will be able to position themselves somewhere on a spectrum ranging from being almost totally risk averse to dare-devil. Measuring the part of people's personality associated with their risk taking behaviour, 'risk propensity', however remains notoriously problematic (Nicholson et al., 2005). Currently there are no reliable or established tools for measuring a person's risk taking behaviour and most methods rely either on people answering a questionnaire or responding to a series of hypothetical situations that are put to them. Most modern attempts at measuring risk propensity try to separate out various domains in which a person might take or avoid risks.

Common health-related risk taking might involve smoking or alcohol use and people in contemporary society are at liberty to choose whether to indulge in these behaviours – or not – despite the implications for the future use of health services. People with long-term conditions, however, may find that sanctions are imposed on them if they 'persist' in taking risk related decisions that are deemed to be harmful for them.

The assessment of risk

Prediction is very difficult, especially about the future. (Niels Bohr)

A large component of professional life is implicitly or explicitly concerned with the assessment of risk; a fire officer will make a judgement about possible fire hazards; a police officer makes risk assessments all the time about possible dangers in an incident; teachers are wondering how risky particular activities might be for the young people in their charge; finance workers are assessing the risk of monetary gains or losses, etc. Lay people including people with long-term conditions also take decisions based on their own, informal risk assessments throughout their lives: Should I continue to take my medication? Can I go on holiday away from my usual support networks? Should I continue to smoke even though my breathing seems to be getting worse? Perhaps I could have a drink – even though I am taking antibiotics?

Professional risk assessment is usually not done by people affected by that risk and the relationship between risk-assessor and risk-taker is critical to the process. Sven Hansson, a Swedish professor of philosophy, succinctly expresses the problem: 'risks are inextricably connected with interpersonal relationships. They do not just "exist"; they are taken, run or imposed' (2002: 25). Professional attempts at risk assessment always involve a difference in status and power between those making the assessment and those affected by the decisions based on that risk assessment for whom the decisions may have a major effect.

There is a trend for health and social care organizations, and indeed most other public bodies, to veer towards risk aversion in order to reduce the possibility of legal action for negligence or formal inquiries into their professional practice. The proliferation of risk assessment forms and possibly over-zealous processes reflects the need for organizations to protect themselves from legal action, and also indicates anxiety amongst professionals keen to avoid being the focus of inquiry into bad practice. This negative conceptualization of risk is associated with defensive practices amongst professionals and organizations. Decisions may tend to focus on the need to avoid risk altogether and 'cover our backs' which at an institutional level is sometimes called 'reputational risk management'.

Individual health and social care workers working within this risk avoidance culture, may feel compelled to pressurize people who use their services into reducing their risks. In any event it is hard for health and social care workers to avoid the burden of paperwork and the bureaucratization of risk assessment procedures.

Professional risk assessment

The two main professional approaches to risk assessment are usually labelled as 'clinical' and 'actuarial' although in practice the techniques may well overlap and both may be used together. An actuary is an expert in statistics, usually someone who calculates insurance risks. In health and social care contexts the actuarial approach is one adopted by professionals who have access to statistical information on particular populations, for example people of a certain age, or who have been diagnosed with particular conditions. By looking at collective data it is hoped that the possibility or probability of an adverse event for individuals can be estimated (Kemshall, 2007). Unfortunately the instruments that have so far been designed to calculate risk on an actuarial basis remain imperfect:

> Our analyses indicated that two popular ARAIs (actuarial risk assessment instruments) used in risk assessment have poor precision. The margins of error for risk estimates made using the tests were substantial, even at the group level. At the individual level the margins of error were so high as to render the test results virtually meaningless. (Hart et al., 2007: s63)

Actuarial models of risk assessment may be attractive to planners and managers of services because they appear to offer a technical and 'objective' means of assessing risk. However it is always important to question the validity and comparability of the research studies on which the calculations are based (Silver and Miller, 2002). There is also a problem with attempting to transfer the aggregated risk factors based on group, statistical information to an individual situation. For example if actuarial assessment indicates that a person with a particular cancer has a six in ten chance of surviving five years there is no simple guidance that will tell you whether the individual will be in the 60 percent survival group – or not (Kemshall, 2007).

The clinical approach

Risk assessments based on a clinical approach with people who have long-term mental health issues in their lives are based on the professional's knowledge of the individual's past and present behaviour and their current state of mental health. The professional workers will review this information through the lens of their own previous experience and training. For example a mental health worker might learn that the individual in front of them is hearing voices that appear to be giving them instructions about self harm. Further evidence may be gained from reading past clinical notes prepared by other health workers who have recorded previous episodes when self harm has been considered or attempted. In this way layers of evidence are obtained and an assessment is made on the likelihood of self harm for this individual. However this approach is not without its own problems. Often the focus on risks may tend to encourage practitioners to 'look for what is going wrong, rather than what is going right' (Booth and Booth, 1998). A hazard-based approach may severely restrict the activities of people being assessed. This restriction may affect the quality of life of the restricted person much more than running the risk of a potential hazard in the future ... which may of course never happen:

> If agencies and their employees take a narrow hazard approach to risk, they will contribute to the disempowerment of people. (Alaszewski and Alaszewski, 2002: 62)

All professional work ultimately contains a subjective element and perceptual bias remains a problem (Ward and Eccleston, 2000). Research by Spengler at al. (2009) suggests that clinical approaches to risk assessment may have problems associated with limited accuracy and that even experience does not always lead to improved judgement. Indeed assessors working as health and social care practitioners may base their decisions or recommendations on their experience of other people they have encountered in similar situations rather than on more objective or nuanced evidence regarding the person who is currently being assessed:

> Given that clinical realities increasingly require risk assessments, it is an ongoing challenge to implement such less-than-perfect structured risk assessment methods into clinical practice and cautiously handle the balance between predictive nihilism – 'nothing works' – and predictive over-enthusiasm – 'decisions are close to perfection'. (Bengtson and Langstrom, 2007: 151)

More recently a holistic approach that combines actuarial and clinical types of assessment is commonly advocated and applied in practice (Buchanan, 2008; Titterton, 2004).

A holistic approach based on 'critical practice' will encourage workers to see risk assessment more as a tool that complements professional judgement rather than as an end in itself (Munro, 2004). In practice most experienced health and social care practitioners will use a mixture of assessment approaches and will explicitly or implicitly use a combination of their own clinical experience, the skills and knowledge that they have learned from other members of their team and wisdom gained from research literature and theoretical publications. Reliance on a single assessment process might be considered unduly rigid and create problems.

Vulnerability and the right to take risks

Although many organizations and institutions working in the field of health and social care place emphasis on the vulnerability of the people with long-term conditions they care for and hence on protection and minimizing risk for them, this can raise some uncomfortable issues. Perhaps this approach represents a step backwards towards a patronizing model of care and away from user-led and empowering services? When people choose to accept risks in their lives, for example when they decide to stay living independently in a house that is familiar but which could be considered 'risky' perhaps it is their right to decide where to draw the line? There remains a tension between the need for protection and the need to respect diversity, identity and individual autonomy. Clearly not all people who use mental health services want to be protected and have their 'risks' assessed. The disabled people's movement has led the way and remains adamant that discrimination, in terms of access to basic resources such as housing, transport, income and assistance, creates situations in which people are made vulnerable. For example the basic design of housing or workplaces can make their use by people with physical impairments impossible (EDF, 1999).

The notion of vulnerability is itself associated with considerable complexity. The term 'vulnerable' could be applied to a broad group of people who may be potential or actual users of health or social care services. It may also be applied in law to people who are lacking the capacity to take decisions on their own behalf (Department of Health, 2005), or who are unable to manage their own affairs. But should it also be applied to people who are usually able to manage their affairs but who find themselves in unsafe situations perhaps because of a long-term medical condition or disability?

Some people may internalize a sense of vulnerability and come to view themselves as unable to cope with everyday situations. Vulnerability is not a fixed state and as conditions improve or worsen, or when support is offered or withdrawn, people can feel more or less vulnerable.

Risk and society

The 'risk society thesis' is associated with the work of Ulrich Beck (1992), a German sociologist, who looked at the changes within society during the twentieth century and considered that risk is inherent in the changes associated with modern life. As societies have developed and evolved away from traditional forms of organization new mega-dangers or hazards have emerged. In Beck's opinion these risky features have relatively recently been created by society itself, but appear to be no longer manageable within any individual's capacity to effect change or realistically protect themselves. Contemporary society might appear to be characterized by risk and the debates on how it should be managed at personal and institutional levels. In the health and social care context it is clear that people expect the state to protect its citizens from risk, but this protection itself may be considered stigmatizing, patronizing or excessively restrictive.

During the early days of the Welfare State an expectation developed that some form of social or health related assistance would provide individual members of society with an almost universal safety net. People came to expect to be looked after in their time of need — whatever the cost to society. Kemshall (2007) has proposed that this expectation of 'welfare society' has largely been replaced by a more manageable 'risk society' in which preoccupations with need have been replaced by the language of risk. Services that might have once been universal now have to be restricted and rationed according to risk criteria ... people at greatest risk, or those posing the greatest risk, will be considered for services and state provided interventions. This shift in emphasis has not been restricted to social service or welfare provision but is also apparent in the criminal justice system and within the health service itself. The work of social workers is often focused around 'risk assessment' and the consideration of 'bad risk'. How likely is it that this person will harm themselves, how possible is it that this person will harm other people?

At the end of the Second World War a general consensus developed in many western societies determined to develop ways in which every citizen could benefit from the growth and development of that society. Avoidance or minimization of risk was one of the dominant features of social policy at that time. People would be protected from harm as much as possible if they became ill, lost their jobs, needed housing or when they were too old to work. In the UK this social imperative was developed as the Welfare State and was most comprehensively expressed as government policies that followed the publication of the Beveridge Report (Abel-Smith, 2007):

> The object of government in peace and in war is not the glory of rulers or of races but the happiness of the common man … the purpose of victory is to live into a better world than the old world. (Beveridge, 1942: 171)

The grand language of the Beveridge Report reflected a desire to minimize or avoid risk and for the state to provide the means for doing this. The much quoted phrase from *'from cradle to grave'* encapsulates the desire to shield people from risk throughout the course of their life. The quest for universal provision of health and welfare services has been eroded over the intervening period by a number of factors and many people – particularly in times of financial stringency – continue to question whether such universal government sponsored intervention is ever possible or indeed desirable (Giddens, 1998).

Suicide and self harm risk assessment

A balance between individual and collective concerns about risk is particularly played out in the field of mental health. Professional concern is triggered if the person who is going through a period of mental distress is considered to be a danger to themselves – and of course enormous social, professional and especially political concern is aroused if the person is considered to be a danger to other people in the wider community.

How can a person be assessed to see whether they may be at risk of harming themselves, or even taking their own life? This is a continuing challenge to health and social care workers and even the most experienced practitioners find this situation to be one of the most complex aspects of their work with potentially vulnerable people. There is no substitute for health and social care workers developing a relationship with the person being assessed and listening to them talk about their thoughts and feelings. However, some actuarial assessments are possible based on the way that people in similar situations have behaved previously. Dag Tidemalm and his colleagues in Sweden (2008) followed up almost 40,000 people for 30 years who had previously attempted suicide. They found that having a specific diagnosed mental health problem was a strong predictor of 'successful' or 'completed' suicide at a later date. The strongest predictors were a diagnosis of schizophrenia or bipolar disorder. Gunnell et al. (2008) followed up 75,000 people discharged from psychiatric inpatient care in England. They found that almost 5,000 of these people were readmitted to hospital for self harm within one year of discharge, one third of these within one month of the original discharge. The most common diagnostic categories that indicated a high risk of future self harm included 'personality disorder', depression, anxiety and substance misuse.

Dangerousness

Exploring the complex link between mental distress and violent behaviour is fraught with difficulty. Publicity relating to people who have been experiencing mental turmoil and who have become violent is frequently portrayed in the media. This exposure has affected the way that the general public and policy makers think about, and fear, people with mental health issues in their lives. Mental health legislation in almost every country includes what is known as an obligatory dangerousness criterion (ODC). An ODC provides the force of the law behind treatment without consent to people in mental distress if they are deemed to be a risk to themselves or others. Some commentators feel that the use of the law in this way unfairly discriminates against the vast majority of people in mental distress who will never become violent (Large et al., 2008):

> Dangerousness criteria unfairly discriminate against the mentally ill, as they represent an unreasonable barrier to treatment without consent, and they spread the burden of risk that any mentally ill person might become violent across large numbers of mentally ill people who will never become violent. (Large et al., 2008: 877)

People who are in the midst of a period of mental distress do, on occasion, become violent, but recent reviews (Choe et al., 2008) have shown that they are greatly outnumbered by those who are the subjects of violence rather than the perpetrators. Brekke and colleagues (2001) found that among people living in the community who had been given the label of 'schizophrenia', 6.4% had contact with the police for alleged 'aggression against others' in the past three years while 34.0% reported being violently victimized themselves. Wider epidemiological surveys of the whole population, not just those who have been given a mental illness diagnosis back up this finding. American surveys found that 3% of people without a mental health diagnosis reported being a victim of violence in the previous year compared with 25% of those deemed to have a 'severe mental illness' (Teplin et al., 2005). One USA study found that mental illness only contributed 2% to the total violence experienced in that country (Corrigan and Watson, 2005).

Sometimes people internalize potential problems and believe for themselves the negative stereotypes prevalent in the media:

'I would love to go out more places such as the local pub and library but am too frightened to in case I am dangerous. I have never been dangerous but you read about schizophrenics being dangerous all the time in the paper, so I thought that because I have schizophrenia that I would be dangerous if I went out.' (Danny, Ayr)

'If someone is stabbed in the street then it's automatically one of us! They think we get off lightly with a shorter jail sentence. I really find this disheartening; it makes you go into your shell, which makes things worse. Then you get a fear of going out in case you get insulted, and the violence which may accompany – oh my god!' (Gregor, Western Isles)
    See Me Project 2009

But some people in the midst of, or as part of, their mental distress do commit acts of violence and this contributes to the negative stereotypes and problematic public perception of all people with mental health issues in their lives (Hinshaw and Stier, 2008; Link et al., 1999).

The intricate link between violence and mental distress has been further explored by Eric Elbogen and Sally Johnson (2009), American forensic psychiatry researchers. They used a survey of almost 35,000 people to attempt to determine what features might predict violent behaviour. Detailed analysis of this sample revealed that severe mental illness alone did not predict future violence. However, violence was associated with historical (past violence, juvenile detention, physical abuse, parental arrest), clinical (substance abuse, perceived threats), dispositional (age, sex, income) and contextual (recent divorce, unemployment, victimization) factors. People with mental health issues in their lives had more of these things happening to them:

    … people with mental illness did report violence more often, largely because they showed other factors associated with violence. Consequently, understanding the link between violent acts and mental disorder requires consideration of its association with other variables such as substance abuse, environmental stressors, and history of violence. (Elbogen and Johnson, 2009:152)

Managing the risk of dangerousness

There is enormous pressure on mental health workers to make sure that the people they are responsible for don't become a danger to others in wider society. Much mental health legislation is designed in an attempt to keep 'dangerous mental health patients' off the streets. The political imperative to protect members of the general public is enormous and influences the way that mental health systems are organized (Kemshall, 2009). But how can mental health workers predict who might pose a risk and become violent to other people?

> Using clinical judgment alone, mental health professionals cannot predict individual patient violence much more accurately than chance. (Swanson, 2008: 191)

Some additional features in peoples' lives can be used as pointers to possible future violence; just having a mental health diagnosis is not sufficient (Woods and Lasiuk, 2008). For example people who have been given the psychiatric label 'schizophrenia', and who are also illicit substance abusers do have an increased risk of committing violent crime. A research study in Sweden (Fazel et al., 2009), showed that this combination of 'co-morbidities' was quite a good predictor of violent crime – 27% of people with both these diagnoses committed a violent offence at some time.

Jeffrey Swanson, the American medical sociologist, claims that clinicians and people responsible for managing the risk of possible violence amongst people with mental health issues in their lives should consider the wider picture:

> We have large numbers of people with severe mental illness living in jails, homeless shelters, and substandard apartments in impoverished neighbourhoods where every block has two liquor stores and a pawn shop. Then we talk about preventing violence by tweaking antipsychotic treatment regimes. (Swanson, 2008: 191)

Individual practitioners working with people who are going through periods of mental distress as well as those in contact with people with other long-term conditions are under scrutiny from the organizations that employ them and from the media to not make mistakes when it comes to risk taking. There certainly appears to be a paradox in the way that much of the media portrays the subject of risk in the sphere of health and social care. On the one hand those in control of broadcast and written media seem to recognize that dramatic stories of 'risk gone wrong' are a staple for widespread publicity and are enjoyed by the general public. Shocking stories of abuse and neglect seem to sell newspapers and produce good viewing figures. The general public appears to be fascinated by graphic details and prurient, vicarious information. When there is someone within a professional group apparently to blame for a scandal the media often seem to rush to judgement. The competence of entire professional groups, for example social workers or probation officers, is often called into question because of isolated cases of poor judgement or unsatisfactory care.

Of course when an official enquiry does find fault with individuals or health and social care services the media can be merciless in relaying the criticism without any attempt to provide balance to the story or discuss possible extenuating circumstances. On the other hand the media often seems quick to call into question any measures that may be taken to protect vulnerable individuals and communities 'Protect us from the "Nanny State", … this is Health and Safety gone mad!' Modern professionals are now mainly resigned to the fact that their decisions and motives may well come under scrutiny and be subject to media attention and that they may have to act in a defensive manner.

Summary

Professionals in the health and social care arena often find themselves having to make risk assessments, the results of which may have serious consequences for people with long-term conditions who are having their risks assessed. The process of making a risk assessment epitomizes and emphasizes the power differential between 'client' and 'professional'. Risk assessments can never be considered to be objective, value neutral or even particularly accurate, but have become a central part of the way that people with 'needs' are judged and controlled by those in charge of resources. This chapter has looked particularly at people who are going through periods of significant mental distress, but similar concerns and considerations are shared with making risk assessments on people with many other long-term conditions.

Further reading

Beck, U. (1992) *Risk Society: Towards a New Modernity*. Newbury Park, CA: Sage.

Hansson, S. (2002) 'Philosophical perspectives on risk', keynote address at the Research in Ethics and Engineering conference, Delft University of Technology, April. [Online] Available at: http://www.infra.kth.se/~soh/PhilPerspRisk-text.pdf (accessed 3 November 2010).

Kemshall, H. (2009) 'Mental health, mental disorder, risk and public protection', in J. Reynolds, R. Muston, T. Heller, J. Leach, M. McCormick, J. Wallcraft and M. Walsh (eds), *Mental Health Still Matters*. Basingstoke: Palgrave Macmillan.

Neuberger, J. (2008) *Unkind, Risk Averse and Untrusting – If This Is Today's Society, Can We Change It?* London: Joseph Rowntree Foundation. [Online] Available at: http://www.jrf.org.uk/sites/files/jrf/2280.pdf (accessed 3 November 2010).

Woods, P. and Lasiuk, G. (2008) 'Risk prediction: A review of the literature', *Journal of Forensic Nursing*, 4: 1–11.

Zuckerman, M. (2006) *Sensation Seeking and Risky Behaviour*. Washington: American Psychological Association.

References

Abel-Smith, B. (2007) 'The Beveridge Report: its origins and outcomes', *International Social Security Review*, 45: 5–16.

Alaszewski, A. and Alaszewski, H. (2002) 'Toward the creative management of risk: Perceptions, practices and policies', *British Journal of Learning Disabilities*, 30: 56–62.

Beck, U. (1992) *Risk Society: Towards a New Modernity*. Newbury Park, CA: Sage.

Bengtson, S. and Langstrom, N. (2007) 'Unguided clinical and actuarial assessment of re-offending risk: A direct comparison with sex offenders in Denmark', *Sex Abuse*, 19: 135–53.

Beveridge, W. (1942) *Social Insurance and Allied Services*. Cmd. 6404. London: HMSO.

Booth, T. and Booth, W. (1998) *Growing Up with Parents who have Learning Difficulties*. London: Routledge.

Brekke, J., Prindle, C. and Bae, S. (2001) 'Risk for individuals with schizophrenia who are living in the community', *Psychiatric Services*, 52: 1358–66.

Buchanan, A. (2008) 'Risk of violence by psychiatric patients: Beyond the "actuarial versus clinical" assessment debate', *Psychiatric Services*, 59: 184–90.

Choe, J., Teplin, L. and Adra, K. (2008) 'Perpetration of violence, violent victimization, and severe mental illness: Balancing public health concerns', *Psychiatric Services*, 59: 153–64.

Corrigan, P. and Watson, A. (2005) 'Findings from the National Co-morbidity Survey on the frequency of violent behaviour in individuals with psychiatric disorder', *Psychiatry Research*, 136: 153–62.

Department of Health (2005) *Mental Capacity Act 2005*. London: Department of Health.

EDF (European Disability Forum) (1999) *How Article 13 Disability Directives Can Combat Disability Discrimination*, EDF 99/3.

Elbogen, E. and Johnson, S. (2009) 'The intricate link between violence and mental disorder', *Archives of General Psychiatry*, 66: 152–61.

Fazel, S., Langstrom, N., Hjern, A., Grann, M. and Lichtenstein, P. (2009) 'Schizophrenia, substance abuse and violent crime', *JAMA*, 301: 2016–23.

Giddens, A. (1998) *The Third Way*. Cambridge: Polity.

Gunnell, D., Hawton, K., Ho, D., Evans, J., O'Connor, S., Potokar, J., Donovan, J. and Kapur, N. (2008) 'Hospital admissions for self harm after discharge from psychiatric inpatient care: Cohort study', *British Medical Journal*, 337: a2278.

Hansson, S. (2002) 'Philosophical perspectives on risk', keynote address at the Research in Ethics and Engineering conference, Delft University of Technology, 25 April. [Online] Available at: http://www.infra.kth.se/~soh/PhilPerspRisk-text.pdf (accessed 3 November 2010).

Hart, S., Michie, C. and Cooke, D. (2007) 'Precision of actuarial risk assessment instruments: Evaluating the "margins of error" of group v. individual predictions of violence', *British Journal of Psychiatry*, 190: s60–5.

Hinshaw, S. and Stier, A. (2008) 'Stigma as related to mental disorders', *Annual Review of Clinical Psychology*, 4: 367–93.

Kemshall, H. (2007) 'Risk assessment and management: An overview', in J. Lishman (ed.), *Handbook for Practice Learning in Social Work and Social Care – Knowledge and Theory*, 2nd edn. London: Jessica Kingsley.

Kemshall, H. (2009) 'Mental health, mental disorder, risk and public protection', in J. Reynolds, R., Muston, T. Heller, J. Leach M. McCormick, J. Wallcraft and M. Walsh (eds), *Mental Health Still Matters*. Basingstoke: Palgrave Macmillan.

Large, M., Ryan, C., Nielssen, O. and Hayes, R. (2008) 'The danger of dangerousness: Why we must remove dangerousness criterion from our mental health acts', *Journal of Medical Ethics*, 34: 877–81.

Link, B., Phelan, J. and Bresnahan, M. (1999) 'Public conceptions of mental illness: Labels, causes, dangerousness, and social distance', *American Journal of Public Health*, 89: 1328–33.

Llewllyn, D. (2008) 'The psychology of risk taking: Towards integration of psychometric and neuropsychological paradigms', *American Journal of Psychology*, 121: 363–76.

Lupton, D. and Tulloch, J. (2002) '"Life would be pretty dull without risk": voluntary risk-taking and its pleasures', *Health, Risk and Society*, 4: 113–24.

Munro, E. (2004) 'A simpler way to understand the results of risk assessment instruments', *Children and Youth Services Review*, 26: 873–83.

Neuberger, J. (2008) *Unkind, Risk Averse and Untrusting – If This is Today's Society, Can We Change It?* London: Joseph Rowntree Foundation. [Online] Available at: http://www.jrf.org.uk/sites/files/jrf/2280.pdf (accessed 3 November 2010).

Nicholson, N., Soane, E., Fenton-O'Creevy, M. and Willman, P. (2005) 'Personality and domain-specific risk taking', *Journal of Risk Research*, 8: 157–76.

See Me Project (2009) *Media Guidelines: A Practical Guide for Stigma Stop Watchers*. Available at: www.seemescotland.org.uk/positivereporting/mediaguidelinesforstigmastopwatchers (accessed 27 July 2011).

Silver, E. and Miller, L. (2002) 'A cautionary note on the use of actuarial risk assessment tools for social control', *Crime and Delinquency*, 48: 138–61.

Spengler, P., White, M., Aegisdottir, S. and Maugherman, A. (2009) 'The meta-analysis of clinical judgement project: Effects of experience on judgment accuracy', *The Counseling Psychologist*, 37: 350–99.

Swanson, J. (2008) 'Prediction versus prevention: Predicting the unpredicted: Managing violence risk in mental health care', *Psychiatric Services*, 59: 191–3. [Online] Available at: http://psychservices.psychiatryonline.org/cgi/reprint/59/2/191 (accessed 3 November 2010).

Teplin, L., McClelland, G. and Abram, K. (2005) 'Crime victimization in adults with severe mental illness: Comparison with the National Crime Victimization Survey', *Archives of General Psychiatry*, 62: 911–21.

Tidemalm, D., Langstrom, N., Lichtenstein, P. and Runeson, B. (2008) 'Risk of suicide attempt according to coexisting psychiatric disorded: Swedish cohort study with long-term follow-up', *British Medical Journal*, 337: a2205.

Titterton, M. (2004) *Risk and Risk Taking in Health and Social Welfare*. London: Jessica Kingsley.

Ward, T. and Eccleston, L. (2000) 'The assessment of dangerous behaviour: Research and clinical issues', *Behaviour Change*, 17: 53–68.

Woods, P. and Lasiuk, G. (2008) 'Risk prediction: A review of the literature', *Journal of Forensic Nursing*, 4: 1–11.

Zuckerman, M. (2006) *Sensation Seeking and Risky Behaviour*. Washington: American Psychological Association.

Zuckerman, M. and Kuhlman, D. (2000) 'Personality and risk-taking: common biosocial factors', *Journal of Personality*, 68: 999–1029.

14

What About the Carers?

Mary Larkin

Overview

- Community care
- The effects of caring on carers
- The modernization agenda
- The modernization agenda and carers
- Conclusion

Discussion, debate and policy relating to the management of the complex needs of individuals with long-term conditions often focuses on the formal organization and delivery of health and social care. As a result, the more than significant contribution made by those caring for people with these conditions on an informal basis is often overlooked. The term 'carer' is used to refer to someone caring for a person who cannot care for himself/herself and, excluding benefits, carries this out on an unpaid basis. This chapter focuses on the carers of people with long-term conditions who cannot self-manage, and aims to provide an analysis of the role of unpaid carers in the UK in delivering health and social care for this group of people. It starts with some historical contextualization and outlines the development of community care, as well as showing how this led to both the introduction of the term 'carer' and an increase in the number of carers who care for people with long-term conditions. This will be followed by a discussion of the impact of caring on the lives of these carers. The chapter will then explore subsequent policy developments in community care for people with long-term conditions and the implications of these policy shifts for their carers. The last section will consider the future role of carers in the UK in the delivery of health and social care to people with long-term conditions.

Community care

In order to explore the role of carers in relation to long-term conditions, it is necessary to discuss the concept of 'community care'. This concept can be traced as far back as the early 1900s when the 1904–08 Royal Commission on the Care of the Feeble Minded gave the first indication of a policy shift from institutional to 'community care'. The growing emphasis on 'community care' in policy documents gathered momentum in the 1970s and 1980s, culminating in the National Health Service and Community Care Act 1990 (OPSI, 1990) (implemented in April 1993). Other subsequent legislation which have been influential in progressing 'community care' are the Carers Recognition and Services Act (1995), and the Carers (Equal Opportunities) Act (2004) (Larkin, 2011).

Since the 1970s 'community care' appears to have taken on different meanings in various policy documents. This has led to criticisms that it is yet another 'contested term used by different people in different ways at different points in time' (Means et al., 2008: 3). However, a key theme is that people with chronic illnesses are no longer to be cared for in long-stay hospitals and other types of large institutions. Instead they are to be cared for in their own homes by family members and/or significant others within the community, or in small scale institutions. More specifically, 'community care' has come to be used to describe care for people in need which is based on support and care for individuals in their homes provided through a mixed economy of care. This refers to care that is provided *informally* through the individual and collective efforts of family members and those in the community on an unpaid basis, supported *formally* by paid professionals employed by statutory and voluntary services (Means et al., 2008; Parker, 1985).

Informal care has become central to the delivery of 'community care'. Although people have always cared informally for family and friends, the development of 'community care' has led to the term 'carer' becoming part of the English language (Bytheway and Johnson, 1998; Davey and Popay, 1993). It started to be used in official policy documents, such as the White Paper *Caring for People* (Department of Health, 1989) in the 1980s and around this time 'carers' began to be officially recognized as an identifiable group (Heaton, 1999). However, it was The National Health Service and

Community Care Act 1990 (OPSI, 1990) that legally enshrined the term 'carer' and institutionalized it within social policy. As a consequence of this Act, those already carrying out this role had the opportunity to be recognized as carers and receive support. In addition, increasing numbers of people have found themselves taking on the role of unpaid carer (Brindle, 2001; Dean and Thompson, 1996; Parker and Lawton, 1994).

The political and legal adoption of the concept of 'community care' also heralded a major change in the management of long-term conditions. It meant that those with these conditions who did not require hospitalization could live and receive the care they needed in their own homes rather than residential establishments. As a result, over the past three decades there has been a progressive shift to people with long-term conditions who are unable to self-manage being cared for in their own community. For many people with a long-term condition, the introduction of community care therefore represented greater independence (Blakemore, 2007; Means et al., 2008; Parker, 1985). At the same time there has been a considerable growth in the number of unpaid carers for this group in British society. The increasing numbers of people living with long-term conditions will result in a continued growth in the number of carers. Currently, there are around 5 million carers and analysis suggests that there will be a need for another 3.4 million informal unpaid carers over the next 35 years (Department of Health, 2006; The Health and Social Care Information Centre, 2010a, 2010b; Yeandle et al., 2007).

The effects of caring on carers

Since the emergence of the concept of the 'carer' in the 1980s, research on carers and their experiences has burgeoned. This has drawn upon both primary and secondary data and been carried out at national and local level by a variety of bodies, such as voluntary organizations, government departments and academic institutions. Quantitative and qualitative methods have been used, often in combination. These include surveys with structured questionnaires, individual biographies, and in-depth interviews. Sample sizes and timescales have varied considerably; some have involved an in-depth interview with as few as six carers over the course of one week, others have involved as many as 500 postal interviews over a number of years. Whilst much of the literature is empirical, there have been theoretical analyses of caring too, for example, from feminist and Foucauldian perspectives. The body of research on carers has also been regularly reviewed (Brechin, 1998; Parker, 1985, 1995; Stalker, 2003; Twigg et al., 1990).

Despite its different perspectives and purposes, the literature on caring 'has had an important impact in terms of policy, practice, theory and ethics issues and contributed to the emergence of caring as a significant issue for social policy and practice' (Barnes, 2006: 1). Moreover, it has increased understanding of carers' experiences and the effects of caring on them; caring has been shown to be subject to many variable influences which interact with each other and with external factors to shape each individual carer's experience. Firstly, there is their *diversity* – not only do their social and cultural backgrounds reflect the diversity and demographics of the rest of society but some are also service users themselves. Another influence on caring is the *person being cared for* – this person may be a close family member, a friend or a neighbour. They may be living with a wide range of physical and mental conditions which give rise to complex needs (Barnes, 2006; Pickard et al., 2007; The Health and Social Care Information Centre, 2010a, 2010b). A further variable is the *multifaceted tasks associated with caring*. Examples are practical tasks such as shopping, cooking and cleaning. In addition to these tasks, carers may be required to carry out health care tasks including:

- physical tasks (feeding, washing and toileting), some of which can be physically demanding (lifting and hoisting)
- provision of emotional support, empathy and affection
- administering medication, giving injections, changing dressings and incontinence management
- transporting dependants
- organising services for the cared for person in order to manage their illness (Cancian and Oliker, 1999; Pickard and Glendinning, 2002; Twigg and Atkin, 1994; Seale, 2000).

The variation in the extent to which carers carry out these tasks and the length of time they spend doing them illustrates the complex web of interactions that take place as part of the caring experience. The amount and nature of accessible help available is an important factor in the variations identified. There is also an interaction between the nature of the care recipient's condition and length of time spent caring each week; a person in the early stages of Multiple Sclerosis may only require a few hours of practical support each week. By contrast the carer of someone with advanced Alzheimer's disease, may have to carry out all of the above tasks and devote 50 hours or more per week to caring (Bond et al., 2003; Larkin, 2011; The Health and Social Care Information Centre, 2010a, 2010b).

Thus 'care can be defined by its complexity' (Ray et al., 2009: 115) and being a carer is context specific. Nonetheless, research has shown that there are commonalities in carers' experiences. Carers often choose to care and many see it as a welcome opportunity to undertake a new role. There is evidence that they find caring rewarding, worthwhile and satisfying and that it brings them much joy and gives them a sense of identity. Indeed some have found it to be life changing experience which has improved their relationship with the person for whom they care and influenced their choice of employment post-caring. However, the execution of the role of carer and its associated tasks and responsibilities also place considerable demands on carers. Studies have shown that caring affects physical and psychological health. Carers may experience a wide range of problems such as depression, anxiety, emotional distress, stress, feeling tired, hernias, heart problems, arthritis, asthma, giddiness, backaches, and headaches. Caring may also impact negatively on personal and sexual relationships, employment opportunities, financial and social circumstances, self-confidence, self-esteem and identity (Gilbert et al., 2009; Glendinning et al., 2009; Hirst, 1999, 2003; Lewis and Meredith, 1988; McLaughlin and Ritchie, 1994; Watson and Doyal, 1999; Yeandle et al., 2007).

Other pressures and problems for carers stem from deficiencies in the implementation of 'community care' policies – critics have pointed to failures in interagency working and the poor quality and inflexibility of both the formal and informal services that are available. Moreover, there have been concerns about the informal support available within communities for carers. Many original community care policies seem to characterize communities as being socially cohesive and containing reliable sources of unpaid support. However, living in a community is not always a positive experience; the community may be blighted by social fragmentation, high crime rates, high unemployment and social inequalities. Therefore, the reality of community life can mean that those providing unpaid care for family members with long-term conditions at home do not receive individual and collective support from other community members (Chamberlynne and King, 2000; Crow and Maclean, 2006; Means et al., 2008).

Furthermore, the physical and social limitations of some long-term conditions, such as Alzheimer's disease, place additional demands on their carers. People providing care may need to continually adjust psychologically and partially reshape their daily life, lifestyle, identity and relationship with the cared-for person throughout the time they provide informal care. Most of those who care for older people with long-term conditions are spouses or adult children and are likely to be advancing in years themselves. Spousal carers of older people are usually of a similar age and, increases in longevity mean that many of those adult children caring for the over 85s are also 65 and over. These carers are more likely to have a pre-existing medical condition and many of the negative effects of caring on them are compounded (Bandeira et al., 2007; Bond et al., 2003; Hanratty et al., 2007; Pickard et al., 2007; Social Exclusion Unit, 2005).

Several policy initiatives have attempted to address some of the negative effects of caring on carers. These include the Carers (Equal Opportunities) Act (2004) which extended carers statutory rights to assessment of their own needs. Measures to support carers and safeguard their health and well-being while they carry out their caring responsibilities are included in the National Strategy for Carers (1999) and the Carers and Disabled Children's Act (2000). A second state pension for carers enabling them to build up a second tier pension whilst they are caring was introduced in The Child Support, Pensions and Social Security Act (2000). More recent reforms within social care have moved in the direction of carer empowerment by improving their access to information and by providing them with opportunities to have their perspectives and experiences integrated into service development, delivery and professional training. For example, *Putting People First* (Department of Health, 2007) emphasizes working with users *and* carers, and treating carers as partners in the planning and delivery of services (Dixon, 2009; Hatton et al., 2008; Larkin, 2011). In other developments involving user-led organizations, carers are defined as important stakeholders (Office for Disability Issues, 2007). Professional training now includes involvement of carers 'as partners' in all areas of the social work curriculum as well as 'in Programme management, student assessment and recruitment activities' (Social Care Institute for Excellence, 2009: 1).

National and local organizations supporting and representing the interests of carers also help improve carers' lives. Over the past few years, these organizations have been increasingly involved in campaigning on behalf of carers' needs and they carry out research to inform policy (Baggott, 2004; Brindle, 2001; Clements, 2009). Such research includes the effects of caring on health, employment and caring, and carers' rights. In addition, they provide a range of support for carers. Examples are benefits advice, advocacy services, information about other services, befriending and counselling, carer support groups, training and drop in sessions (http://www.carers.gov.uk; http://www.carers.org). However, many informal carers do not think of themselves as being a 'carer', and do not avail themselves of services aimed at meeting their needs (Ray et al., 2009). Of further concern is that only one in ten carers make use of support services and this figure is even lower for some carers, such as those from ethnic minority groups (Merrell et al., 2006; Pickard et al., 2007).

Bob's story

Bob has attended a Carers Group for a few months. He has been caring for his wife, who has Multiple Sclerosis, for the last 14 years. During the first few years of her illness, they had both been very active in the local branch of the Multiple Sclerosis Society and Bob had enjoyed being events' organiser. However during the past four years her condition has deteriorated and she now only goes out of the house for medical appointments. Their social life has become virtually non-existent and, apart from family members, they have few visitors. Although Bob did not give up working initially, he was unable to progress in his job because of the restrictions his caring responsibilities imposed on the time he could devote to developing his career. Hence their family income remained low and their financial circumstances worsened when he resigned from his job two years ago in order to provide the extra care his wife needed. Since his caring role had started to involve lifting his wife, he has developed a back problem. Whilst he finds caring his wife very satisfying and that it gives him a real sense of purpose, he often feels isolated and had recently started to take medication for mild depression.

One of Bob's reasons for going to the Carers Group was because he lacked friends with whom he could share his experiences of caring. After the first couple of sessions, he found that his many years of caring enabled him to help others in the group. Now a few of them telephone him when they need advice and emotional support. The group leader has also invited him to accompany her to a meeting about social work training at the University in the nearby city. His new-found role as an 'expert' on caring has started to reinforce his sense of identity and he is feeling well enough to consider discussing a reduction in his medication with his GP.

The modernization agenda

Since the late 1990s the quality and type of community care people with long-term conditions receive has been shaped by the modernization agenda. The aims of the reforms introduced within this agenda are to raise standards of public services, improve care, and focus on service users, matching services more closely to their lives (Means et al., 2008). One of the most significant policy trends in the care of those with long-term conditions and their carers is the *move towards the provision of care at home* for people with long-term conditions. This is illustrated in the following quotation:

> ... there has been a marked shift in the location of nursing care in the UK to the community and more particularly the home ... these changes have been supported by a number of clear policy initiatives ... which indicate that the drive towards the home is set to continue. (McGarry, 2008: 83)

Another dimension of the modernization agenda that impacts on people with long-term conditions is the *drive to encourage patient self-care*. An example of such an initiative is the Expert Patient Programme (EPP). The aim of this programme is primarily to enhance the self-management capacities of people with long-term conditions and improve their quality of life. It encourages them to take more control over their health by developing their understanding of their condition so that they can both manage it in partnership with health care professionals and local support networks (Department of Health, 2005; Lorig et al., 2008; Taylor and Bury, 2007). Whilst research has shown that the Expert Patient Programme has met its aims and has become a central element in the management of long-term conditions, both in this country and other countries, less positive outcomes have also been identified. There are concerns that these programmes may not be suitable for all conditions, do not reach minority groups and some patients benefit more than others. In addition, it has been argued that they do not adequately acknowledge the complexities of the experience of long-term conditions and focus on changing the individual rather than addressing the social variables that shape their responses to their illness and the choices they make (Carr et al., 2006; Griffiths et al., 2005; Lorig et al., 2008; Reeves et al., 2008; Rogers et al., 2008).

A further development within the modernization agenda that affects the lives of people with long-term conditions is the introduction of *personalized models of care*. These were outlined in Chapter 10 and, as explained, they aim to increase service users' independence and give both them and their carers more choice and control over the care they receive (Browning, 2007; Department of Health, 2007; Glendinning et al., 2009).

The modernization agenda and carers

The modernization agenda may have brought greater independence and empowerment for people with long-term conditions but it has also been heavily criticized. Some have questioned the principles underlying its policies and suggest that the main driver is the motivation to reduce health care costs (Lorig et al., 2008; Wilson et al., 2007). Whilst there is relatively little research to date about the modernization agenda in relation to carers specifically, commentators have highlighted the fact that the main source of the additional informal health care required by initiatives to provide care at home for people with long-term conditions is informal carers. They argue that this has led to these carers having a greater role than ever before and a commensurate increase in the demands and pressures on them (Hudson,

2005; Rogers et al., 2008). Feminist critiques have also emphasized how the burdens of these developments fall most heavily on women as they are more likely to carry out all types of care and health care within families. In addition, some families (such as one parent families) may find it more difficult to provide the care required (Means et al., 2008; Pickard et al., 2007).

With reference to *personalized models of care*, in the research that has been carried out to date, carers are often incidental to or only part of the main study (Commission for Social Care Inspection, 2009; Edwards and Waters, 2009; Flynn, 2005; Glendinning et al., 2008; Glynn et al., 2008; Pitts et al., 2009; Waters and Hay, 2009). Although findings have therefore been limited, some useful insights have been produced. For example, whilst personalized models of care enable carers to engage in activities of their choice, they spend more time on 'managerial care' as opposed to 'direct "hands-on" care' (Rosenthal et al., 2007: 756; see also Edwards and Waters, 2009 and Glendinning et al., 2009). However, many important issues have yet to be researched. Personalized models have the potential to change aspects of the caring relationship because carers' identities may be constructed and confirmed through the act of caring and the role of carer can be very significant to carers (Graham, 1991; Larkin, 2008, 2009; Ungerson and Kember, 1997). As these models mean that people with long-term conditions can make more decisions about their own care, in some cases there are formal, contractual relationships between the carer and the service user. The effects of these sorts of changes on carers may also be compounded by any misalignments with their own needs. Hence personalized models of care can lead to an erosion of a carer's self-identity and affect the dynamics of the relationship between people living with a long-term condition and their carer.

Conclusion

Carers are the building blocks in the provision of health and social care for people with long-term conditions. The role of carer can significantly affect carers' lives, and there are growing demands on them resulting from initiatives to move care from long-stay hospitals and institutions to the community and from hospital to the home. Whilst the steps that have been taken to address carers' needs are to be welcomed, there remain issues that need to be taken into consideration in the management of people with long-term conditions in the future. Amongst the key issues are the predicted growth in numbers of carers for individuals with a long-term condition because of the epidemiology of long-term conditions and the predicted extension of the trend of providing care at home. In order to ensure the negative experiences of caring for this group are minimized it is as important to continue to strive to meet their needs as it is to meet those for whom they care. Ways of achieving this include:

- further research into the experience of carers of people with long-term conditions and the impact of policy developments
- more targeted support for the most vulnerable carers, such as older carers
- increased recognition of their diverse range of needs that carers may experience
- identification of 'hidden carers'
- development of creative and innovative practice to reach all carers and encourage their use of support and services.

Summary

This chapter has shown how the introduction of community care has led to the development of the concept of the 'carer'. Community care has also resulted in many more of those with long-term conditions being cared for in their own homes and a simultaneous rise in the number of unpaid carers caring for them. Caring has its rewards, but despite policy initiatives to address its adverse effects, it can have many negative impacts on carers' lives. Since the late 1990s, there have been policy developments which mean that carers' roles in the care of people with long-term conditions are both changing and increasing. These developments include the move to provide more care for people with long-term conditions outside hospitals and within the home, and the drive to increase their choice and control over the care they receive. Consideration of the needs of carers should therefore be permanently integrated into policy, practice and research directed at people with long-term conditions.

Further reading

Department of Health (2007) *Putting People First: A Shared Vision and Commitment to the Transformation of Adult Social Care*. London: HMSO.

Larkin, M. (2009) 'Life after caring: The post-caring experiences of former carers', *British Journal of Social Work*, 39(6): 1026–42.

Means, R., Richards, S. and Smith, R. (2008) *Community Care: Policy and Practice*, 4th edn. Basingstoke: Palgrave Macmillan.

References

Baggott, R. (2004) *Health and Health Care in Britain*, 3rd edn. Great Britain: Macmillan Press Ltd.

Bandeira, D.R., Pawlowski, J., Goncalves, T.R., Hilgert, M.C., Bozzetti, M.C. and Hugo, F.N. (2007) 'Psychological distress in Brazilian caregivers of relatives with dementia', *Aging and Mental Health*, 11(1): 14–19.

Barnes, M. (2006) *Caring and Social Justice*. Basingstoke: Palgrave Macmillan.

Blakemore, K. (2007) *Social Policy: An Introduction*, 3rd edn. Buckingham: Open University Press.

Bond, M., Clark, M. and Davies, S. (2003) 'The quality of life of spouse dementia caregivers: Changes associated with yielding to formal care and widowhood', *Social Science and Medicine,* 57: 2385–95.

Brechin, A. (ed.) (1998) *Care Matters. Concepts, Practice and Research in Health and Social Care*. London: Sage.

Brindle, D. (2001) 'Future tense', *Guardian Society*, 19 September: 4.

Browning, D. (2007) *Evaluation of the Self-Directed Support Network: A Review of Progress up to 31st March 2007*. London: in Control Publications.

Bytheway, B. and Johnson, J. (1998) 'The social construction of carers', in A. Symonds and A. Kelly (eds), *The Social Construction of Community Care*. London: Macmillan.

Cancian, F.M. and Oliker, S.J. (1999) *Caring and Gender*. London: Sage.

Carr, J.L. Moffat, J.A.K., Sharp, D.M and Haines, D.R. (2006) 'Is the Pain Stages of Change Questionnaire (PSOCQ) a useful tool for predicting participation in a self-management programme? Further evidence of validity, on a sample of UK pain clinic patients', *BMC Musculoskeletal Disorders*, 7: 101.

Chamberlayne, P. and King, A. (2000) *Cultures of Care: Biographies of Carers in Britain and the two Germanies*. Bristol: The Policy Press.

Clements, L. (2009) *Carers and Their Rights. The Law Relating to Carers*, 3rd edn. London: Carers UK.

Commission for Social Care Inspection (2009) *The State of Social Care in England 2007–08*. London. CSCI.

Crow, G. and Maclean, C. (2006) 'Community' in G. Payne (ed.), *Social Divisions*. Basingstoke: Macmillan.

Davey, B. and Popay, J. (eds) (1993) *Dilemmas in Health Care*. Buckingham: OUP.

Dean, J. and Thompson, D. (1996) 'Fetishizing the family: The construction of the informal carer', in H. Jones and J. Millar (eds), *The Politics of the Family*. Aldershot: Avebury.

Department of Health (1989) *Caring for People*. London: HMSO.

Department of Health (2005) *Supporting People with Long-term Conditions: An NHS and Social Care Model to Support Local Innovation and Integration*. London: HMSO. [Online] Available at: http://www.dh.gov.uk/dr_consum_dh/groups/dh_digitalassets/@dh/@en/documents/digitalasset/dh_4122574.pdf

Department of Health (2006) *Our Health, Our Care, Our Say*. London: HMSO.

Department of Health (2007) *Putting People First: A Shared Vision and Commitment to the Transformation of Adult Social Care*. London: HMSO. [Online] Available at: http://www.dh.gov.uk/en/Publicationsandstatistics/Publications/PublicationsPolicyAndGuidance/DH_081118

Dixon, J. (2009) 'Adopt the personal touch', *The Guardian*, 28 January: 9.

Edwards, T. and Waters, J. (2009) *It's Your Life – Take Control. The Implementation of Self-directed Support in Hertfordshire*. Hertfordshire: Hertfordshire County Council and in Control Partnerships.

Flynn, M. (2005) *Developing the Role of Personal Assistants.* Leeds: Skills for Care.

Gilbert, E., Ussher, J.M. and Hawkins, Y. (2009) 'Accounts of disruptions to sexuality following cancer: The perspective of informal carers who are partners of a person with cancer', *Health,* 13(5): 523–41.

Glendinning, C., Challis, D. Fernandez, J., Jacobs, S., Jones, K., Knapp, M., Manthorpe, G., Moran, N., Netten, A., Stevens, M. and Wilberforce, M. (2008) *Evaluation of the Individual Budgets Pilot Programme: Final Report.* York: Social Policy Research Unit, University of York.

Glendinning, C., Arksey, H., Jon, K., Moran, N., Netten, A. and Rabiee, P. (2009) *The Individual Budgets Pilot Projects: Impact and Outcomes for Carers.* York: Social Policy Research Unit.

Glynn, M., Beresford, P., Bewley, C., Branfield, F., Butt, J., Croft, S., Dattani Pitt, K., Fleming, J., Flynn, R., Parmore, C., Postle, K. and Turner, M. (2008) *Person-centred Support: What Service Users and Practitioners Say.* York: Joseph Rowntree Foundation.

Graham, H. (1991) 'The concept of caring in feminist research: The case of domestic service', *Sociology,* 25 (1), 61– 78.

Griffiths, C., Motlib, J., Azad, A., Ramsay, J., Eldridge, S., Feder, G., Khanem, R., Munni, R., Garrett, M., Turner, A. and Barlow, J. (2005) 'Randomised controlled trial of a lay-led self-management programme for Bangladeshi patients with chronic disease', *British Journal of General Practice,* 55(520): 831–7.

Hanratty, B., Drever, F., Jacoby, A. and Whitehead, M. (2007) 'Retirement age caregivers and deprivation of area of residence in England and Wales', *European Journal of Ageing,* 4(1): 35–43.

Hatton, C., Duffy, S., Waters, J., Senker, J., Crosby, N., Poll, C., Tyson, A., Towell, D. and O'Brien, J. (2008) *An Evaluation of and Report on in Control's Work 2005–2007.* London: *in Control* Publications.

Heaton, J. (1999) 'The gaze and visibility of the carer: a Foucauldian analysis of the discourse of informal care.' *Sociology of Health and Illness,* 21(6): 759–77.

Hirst, M. (1999) *Informal Care-giving in the Life Course.* York: SPRU.

Hirst, M. (2003) 'Caring-related inequalities in psychological distress in Britain during the 1990s', *Journal of Public Health Medicine,* 25(4): 336–43.

Hudson, B. (2005) 'Sea change or quick fix? Policy on long-term conditions in England', *Health and Social Care in the Community,* 13(4): 378–85.

Larkin, M. (2008) 'Group support during caring and post-caring – the role of carers groups', *Groupwork,* 17(2): 28–51.

Larkin, M. (2009) 'Life after caring: The post-caring experiences of former carers', *British Journal of Social Work,* 39(6): 1026–42.

Larkin, M. (2011) *Social Aspects of Health, Illness and Healthcare: A Handbook.* London: McGraw-Hill.

Lewis, J. and Meredith, B. (1988) *Daughters who Care.* London: Routledge.

Lorig, K.R., Ritter, P.L., Dost, A., Plant, K., Laurent, D.D. and McNeil, I. (2008) 'The expert patients programme online, a 1-year study of an Internet-based self-management programme for people with long-term conditions', *Chronic Illness,* 4(4): 247–56.

McGarry, J. (2008) 'Defining roles, relationships, boundaries and participation between elderly people and nurses within the home: An ethnographic study', *Health and Social Care in the Community,* 17(1): 83–91.

McLaughlin, E. and Ritchie, J. (1994) 'Legacies of caring: The experiences and circumstances of ex-carers', *Health and Social Care*, 2(4): 241–53.

Means, R., Richards, S. and Smith, R. (2008) *Community Care: Policy and Practice,* 4th edn. Basingstoke: Palgrave Macmillan.

Merrell, J., Kinsella, F., Murphy, F., Philpin, S., and Ali, A. (2006) 'Accessibility and equity of health and social care services: Exploring the views and experiences of Bangladeshi carers in South Wales, UK', *Health and Social Care in the Community*, 14(3): 197–205.

Office for Disability Issues (2007) *Annual Report*. London: Office for Disability Issues.

Office of Public Sector Information (1990) *National Health Service and Community Care Act 1990 (c. 19)*. London: HMSO. [Online] Available at: http://www.opsi.gov.uk/ACTS/acts1990/ukpga_19900019_en_2

Parker, G. (1985) *With Due Care and Attention: A Review of Research on Informal Care*. London: FPSC.

Parker, G. (1995) *Where Next for Research on Carers?* Leicester: Nuffield Community Care Studies Unit, University of Leicester.

Parker, G. and Lawton, D. (1994) *Different Types of Care, Different Types of Carer: Evidence from the General Household Survey*. Social Policy Research Unit: HMSO.

Pickard, L. and Glendinning, C. (2002) 'Comparing and contrasting the role of family carers and nurses in the domestic health of frail older people', *Health and Social Care in the Community*, 10(3): 144–50.

Pickard, L., Wittenberg, R., Comas-Herrera, A., King, D. and Malley, J. (2007) 'Care by spouses, care by children: Projections of informal care for older people in England to 2031', *Social Policy and Society*, 6(3): 353–66.

Pitts, J., Soave, V. and Waters, J. (2009) *Doing it Your Way. The Story of Self-directed Support in Worcestershire*. Worcestershire: Worcestershire County Council and *in Control* Partnerships.

Ray, M., Bernard, M. and Phillips, J. (2009) *Critical Issues in Social Work with Older People*. Basingstoke: Palgrave Macmillan.

Reeves, D., Kennedy, A.P., Fullwood, C., Bower, P., Gardner, C., Gately, C., Lee, V., Richardson, G. and Rogers, A.E. (2008) 'Predicting who will benefit from an Expert Patients Programme self-management course', *British Journal of General Practice*, 58(548): 198–203.

Rogers, A., Kennedy, A., Bower, P., Gardner, C., Gately, C., Lee, V., Reeves, D. and Richardson, G. (2008) 'The United Kingdom Expert Patients Programme: Results and implications from a national evaluation', *The Medical Journal of Australia*, 189 (10 Suppl): S21–4.

Rosenthal, C.J., Martin-Matthews, A. and Keefe, J.M. (2007) 'Care management and care provision for older relatives amongst employed informal care-givers', *Ageing and Society*, 27: 755–78.

Seale, C. (2000) 'Changing patterns of death and dying', *Social Science and Medicine*, 51(6): 917–30.

Social Care Institute for Excellence (2009) *Building User and Carer Involvement in Social Work Education*. [Online] available at: http://www.scie.org.uk/publications/ataglance/ataglance19.asp

Social Exclusion Unit (2005) *Excluded Older People. Social Exclusion Unit Interim Report*. Great Britain: Office of the Deputy Prime Minister.

Stalker, K. (ed.) (2003) *Reconceptualising Work with Carers: New Directions for Policy and Practice*. London: Jessica Kingsley.

Taylor, D. and Bury, M. (2007) 'Chronic illness, expert patients and care transition', *Sociology of Health and Illness*, 29(1): 27–45.

The Health and Social Care Information Centre (2010a) *The Survey of Carers in Households – 2009/10 England – Provisional Results*. [Online] Available at: www.ic. nhs.uk/pubs/carersurvey0910

The Health and Social Care Information Centre (2010b) *Personal Social Services Survey of Adult Carers in England – 2009–10*. [Online] Available at: www.ic.nhs.uk/pubs/ psscarersurvey0910

Twigg, J. and Atkin, K. (1994) *Carers Perceived. Policy and Practice in Informal Care*. Buckingham: OUP.

Twigg, J., Atkin, K. and Perring, C (1990) *Carers and Services. A Review of Research*. London: HMSO.

Ungerson, C. and Kember, M. (1997) *Women and Social Policy. A Reader*. Basingstoke: Macmillan.

Waters, J. and Hay, M. (2009) *Steering My Own Course. The Introduction of Self-directed Support in Cambridgeshire*. Cambridgeshire: Cambridgeshire County Council and *in Control* Partnerships.

Watson, S. and Doyal, L. (1999) *Engendering Social Policy*. Great Britain: OUP.

Wilson, P.M., Kendall, S. and Brooks, F. (2007) 'The Expert Patients Programme: A paradox of patient empowerment and medical dominance', *Health and Social Care in the Community*, 15(5): 426–38.

Yeandle, S., Bennett, C., Buckner, L., Fry, G. and Price, C. (2007) *Diversity in Caring: Towards Equality for Carers*. London: Carers UK.

15

Ethics and Long-term Conditions: A Reflective Approach

Stephen Pattison

Overview

- This ethical reflection is based around the question: Are there ways that people can prepare themselves in case they develop a long-term condition in the future?
- Patience, realism, acceptance of limitations and the ability to find possibilities for pleasure within a restricted lifestyle all seem to be pre-requisites for making the best of a long-term condition
- These are precisely the values that are least likely to be learnt within a contemporary society that so highly regards and rewards individualism and the pursuit of wealth
- Some individuals seem naturally suited to, or have learnt how to develop individual characteristics, that make living with a long-term condition tolerable. Others struggle to come to terms with their situation
- Can a study of ethics, in particular the ethics of virtue, help people negotiate or prepare for life with a long-term condition?

Life, some wiseacres say, is a terminal disease. This rather cynical cliché embodies an important insight. That is that life is a very mixed experience of joy, suffering, activity, passivity, expected pleasure, unexpected pain. It is not, as you might say, a bed of roses – for anyone.

And that is an important place to start thinking about the ethics of long-term conditions, illnesses and distress. Indeed, for thinking about anything of importance in human existence.

Ethics is variously understood. It would be possible to dwell at length on the inequity of resource allocation and provision for people with long-term conditions and to make a case for more State support for research and care. I could spend a long time discussing principles of justice and distribution. Or, perhaps more usefully, talk about the ways in which people who live with long-term conditions should be treated by professionals and carers and treat those professional carers in return. It would be possible to discuss social views and barriers to understanding and helping those with long-term conditions so that they are better included in society.

All of these are substantive areas of ethical concern. But instead of considering principles, policies, procedures, prejudices and practices, all central to ethics, I would like to turn to a different way of thinking about ethics and consider the ethics of virtue or character and how they might impinge on our understandings of long-term conditions in society. How might we prepare ourselves for living with long-term conditions either in ourselves or others? What sort of people do we need to become, individually and corporately, to be better prepared for the reality of living with long-term conditions which for many of us are inevitable, even if, or especially if, they come towards the end of our lives? This is a big question and one that is seldom asked amidst the rightly very practical but instrumental needs and concerns of everyday care and concern for those living with long-term conditions. But as individuals most of us will find it hard to avoid it because it has been calculated that 15.4 million people in England currently live with a long-term condition (Kings Fund, 2010). This is about one in three of the total population – and of course this proportion rises with age. So by the time we get to be 65 years old approximately 60% of us will be considered to have a long-term condition of some sort.

I will discuss a bit more about virtue ethics and the ethics of character later, but first let me tell you how I came to think of this as an important issue via a personal story.

A personal story

My friend Donald, who recently died at the age of 84, was a successful academic who throughout his life was a prolific writer. Indeed, his last book, written with the help of a carer who typed out the words, was published just a month before his death. Nothing particularly noteworthy there – academics often keep writing till they die (and not always well!). But there is something noteworthy about this particular man. In the first place, he developed Poliomyelitis in his teens which had distorted his spine and given him chronic health problems throughout his life. He had particular difficulty with breathing. And secondly, for the last five years of his life he became blind. Add to this the fact that he had had a number of strokes in the last few years of his life and was both house- and wheelchair-bound for three years and the book writing begins to sound quite remarkable. Indeed, my own belief is that when he felt that he would no longer write another word, he gave up the will to live.

Donald was a proud, sharp, witty, and articulate man, fully and rightly aware of his own brilliance, who did not suffer fools gladly, though he was generally very kind to those who were just ignorant. A gifted teacher, he had travelled all over the world to attend conferences and had a very outward looking perspective on life. He loved meeting new people and seeing new places.

So I was surprised when, as his health and mobility declined drastically, to discover a 'new' Donald, a man who seemed extraordinarily patient with his condition, was extremely kind and appreciative to all his carers and visitors, and who bore the limits of his very restricted situation with what can only be described as grace. I searched for signs of the frustration, impatience and anger of which I had been the butt very occasionally. I did not find them. I thought about how, if I were in his dependent situation, I would be very angry, very frustrated, very depressed, and very unkind to those around me. I might even try to kill myself. Donald did not seem to manifest many of these symptoms, despite essentially having to suffer the indignities of baby-like dependence. Had he had a personality transplant, or decided to become some kind of saint?

Then it occurred to me that Donald, despite his full and active life, had from a very early age, since he first got Polio, been used to having a restricted life in which he was far more dependent on others than he would have liked. He had long periods of care in hospital in which he had been immobile and at some point in the past he must have made his peace with the limits of that situation and learned the 'virtues' of living with constraint. This did not stop him from living fully and he seldom dwelt upon his skeletal and sight problems, though in fact they consumed a great deal of his time on occasion. Donald would not have been grateful if people had habitually considered him to be a person with special needs, though he was a grateful recipient of discretely offered help if he needed it. Amongst other things, he had filled his mind with reams of poetry that he could recite and think about long after his sight was gone.

Donald did not suffer many of the exacerbating hardships that a lot of people with long-term conditions do. Although he had life-long impairments, he could hold down and do his job (which was compatible with his abilities and needs) and was well paid and resourced. I recount this story about Donald, not because I think he was particularly exceptional, a hero, or a 'celebrity' sufferer, nor a particularly good person, but because I was so impressed by the way in which he lived fully but realistically with his situation until he died. It seemed that he had somehow learned the qualities, attitudes and virtues that allowed him to flourish amidst substantial frustration and restriction, with occasional unpredictable times when he could do more, and many times when he could do less, than he wanted.

Would I be able to do the same? What did Donald have that I have not got? The answer to that appeared to be a set of character dispositions, habits and attitudes to life, such as patience, realism, acceptance of limits, gratitude, seeing the possibilities for pleasure and good within strictly confined situations. In other words, Donald has developed the virtues and character that seemed to allow him to flourish, along with the people around him, as best he and they could.

Why do I not believe myself to possess these very valuable virtues? Perhaps in common with most other people in contemporary society, I have never been encouraged to contemplate acquiring those virtues. Indeed, the values and virtues that Western capitalist society seems to encourage are inimical to living within constraints and valuing dependency in any way (Giddens, 1991, 1992; Lasch, 1991). While I don't want to become President of the USA or the chief executive of a bank, I have been encouraged to think that life is all about being active, making choices, using spending power to having new experiences, achieving ambitions, setting targets, changing to meet new challenges, moving to take new jobs and responsibilities. So the irony would seem to be that people like me, many of us, are brought up to have values, and the virtues that actualize those values, that ill-prepare us for living with long-term conditions of illness, disability, or old age.

Paradoxically, then, increased longevity in our thrusting and developing society means that many more of us are likely to have the opportunity to live with the diminishments of long-term conditions; at the same time, however, we are less well-prepared than we have ever been to cope with them. The learned virtues and habits that make us pleasure-hungry, competitive agents in the market and labour economy are those that are likely to make us feel miserable and useless as the limits and diminishments of old age and long-term conditions encroach. Maybe it is partly because of this mismatch of values and virtues that legalized euthanasia is becoming an increasingly plausible option for those who feel that in terms of the society around them whose norms they have internalized, their lives have no value.

The importance of virtue

Perhaps virtue sounds rather old-fashioned and po-faced in the early twenty-first century, redolent of being good in some rather goody-goody sort of way. It is certainly old-fashioned. Virtue theory is one of the oldest ways of thinking about ethics, originating before Christ in Ancient Greece. It is particularly associated with the so-called 'therapeutic philosophers' and especially with Aristotle. For the therapeutics, philosophy was not just about abstract thinking and being clever with words and concepts (Nussbaum, 1994). Their aim was to help people (upper class men usually) to live full and helpful lives amidst the uncertainties and incurable sufferings of this world. Like Buddhists, many of the therapeutics advocated detachment from earthly bonds, emotions and desires. This was one way of approaching and living with inevitable suffering and loss. The whole of philosophical enquiry and practice was intended to help people to live realistically and fully amidst the constraints of everyday life which was, of course, brief, hard, violent and disease-ridden. Arguably, we need to recover something of this, even in an era of increasing technological mastery and control of the world.

Virtue ethics, currently undergoing a big revival in Western ethical thought, is not so much concerned with how to solve everyday dilemmas or how to use principles appropriately, but more with helping to shape people so that they could achieve their potential (Darwell, 2003; Pence, 1993; Swanton, 2003). The aim of virtuous living is human flourishing, both corporately and for individuals. The big questions for virtue ethics are what sort of world are we trying to shape, and what sort of people do we need to become in order to flourish in that world? There are no questions bigger than these; they are not easy to answer, nor do they have unitary answers upon which everyone can readily agree. However, they do push us beyond just thinking about the next thing that needs to be done. They make us think about what sort of world we want to live in, what will be good for all of us, what sort of values are then needed to make that world a reality, and, crucially, what sort of people we need to be to be able to live in the world both as it is and as it should be.

This is not just an abstract quest. Once we have decided what sort of people we need to be, virtue ethics requires us to identify specific virtues that compose the sort of person we are trying to become. Virtues are morally valuable habits of action, mind and disposition that make up our character and they can be acquired by practice and training. So, for example, we can habituate ourselves to giving money to people on the street as a manifestation of the virtue of generosity.

A virtuous person in any particular context is not then a person who is necessarily outstandingly or heroically good. It is a person who has acquired, perhaps trained themselves in, certain ways of thinking and acting that mean that they hopefully flourish themselves and contribute to the wider flourishing of those around them. Some virtues may be easily acquired by some, e.g. a natural care for others, other virtues may be less easy to gain. But virtue ethicists would argue that in any situation in life there are certain virtues, habits and dispositions that can make a real difference to a person and the people around them.

The sorts of virtues that Aristotle commended were honesty, the pursuit of justice, and courage (Aristotle, 2003). And it is worth noticing in passing that virtues often sit in the middle between possible vices – so, for example, courage sits between, on the one hand, rashness, and on the other, cowardice. Thus the virtues, whichever are adopted and we probably need to think of new ones in the present day, are firmly in the middle ground on sensible, practicable and context-specific actions and attitudes. My friend Donald was neither wholly active nor wholly passive in his diminished state, but rather patiently sought opportunities for pleasure and development where he could find them. Perhaps this represents the virtue of fortitude which lies between pig-headed refusal to accept the limits of the situation and depressed fatalism. He exemplified the virtues that some Christians seek when they pray:

> God, grant me the courage to change the things I can change; the serenity to accept those I cannot change; and the wisdom to know the difference.

Virtues and long-term conditions

This discourse on my friend and an ancient type of ethical thinking may seem a long way from the practicalities of helping people with long-term conditions and those who work with, and make policies, for them. I am also aware that this approach may sound rather passive. Perhaps I am being heard to say that people with long-term conditions and those around them should just console themselves with philosophy and forget about fighting for resources, researching helps and cures, campaigning for justice, and improving life for themselves and those around them.

This is not my intention at all. It is worth remembering that Aristotle and his colleagues formulated their ethical theories in the intensely political and violent world of Greek warrior city states. Their form of ethics was intended to govern social and communal life, not just provide high-minded thoughts for the leisured. Their theories were produced in an era of conflict and strife as well as disease and pestilence so they emerge against a clear background of suffering, discontent and pain. Perhaps that is why courage was such an important virtue in Aristotle's system and it remains so today (Aristotle, 2003). Courage is not just about bearing things, it may be about attack and killing, too!

Another important virtue was that of doing justice. In the present context, virtue ethics in no way brackets out the need for people to create a fair society in which everyone gets their proper share of wealth and resources. In the present context, people who have to live with long-term conditions certainly need this kind of justice, but they perhaps also require the opportunities to contribute fairly to society in such a way that they feel their contributions are valued. This is a highly political and practical matter.

Virtue ethics are not, then, a-political and a-social ethics. They are an ethics about the whole of society, its overall direction and the nature and character of the people who comprise it. They are potentially highly supportive of critics of the status quo.

Western capitalism is rational and instrumental in its approach to life (Ritzer, 2006). This means that people decide what to do consulting their own interests and then they bend the world as far as possible to their will. Its model of humans is that we are atomized psychological individuals who each theoretically have equal rights and are allowed to buy things and sell our labour in the market place (Campbell, 1987; Giddens, 1991). Indeed, our main significance is that we act as consumers and workers; much in our educational and health care systems is provided on the basis that we must be, or become, full players in that market. Unemployment is regarded as a stigmatizing curse that must be eliminated and people who are disabled or unable to participate in the market are thought of as second class, dependent citizens.

The good citizen is one who has a primary loyalty to, and provides for, their employer, themselves, their family and their friends. This person is prepared to move away from those same family and friends if necessary to get work and gain money. S/he, too, has an instrumental, market view of life. S/he cultivates the virtues of autonomy, making personal choices, independence, self-improvement, working hard, economic productivity and detachment from local and familial ties. Schools and universities are seen as providing opportunities for citizens to acquire the proper virtues necessary for what is called full participation in society, but what is actually a very partial engagement of the self in the economy.

I am by no means knocking the society that we have filled with material plenty and technological innovation; this has extended life and opportunities for many, including those with long-term conditions, and also eliminated many kinds of poverty. But in the caricature I have presented here it can be seen that the values and virtues that pertain to market participation are only one way of looking at the world. In some ways, they are individualistic, arbitrary, even tawdry: Where is the big vision of a society that is worth belonging to and where people look after each other instead of seeing others as competitive threats for scarce goods?

This is not a social vision that is going to be much interested in people experiencing long-term conditions that do not generate money either in the market or in the development of treatments. Those with long-term conditions, insofar as they are seen to be outside the market economy, are likely to find that not only are their material needs ignored, but their experience and narratives are seen as irrelevant to common human wisdom and understanding. This is a dangerous exclusion; if we are all connected to each other, we need to learn to live with the intractable and persistent constraints on life and not to imagine that life is one big Disneyland where we can manufacture or purchase pleasure in a pain-free, limit-free existence. (If you want to explore the limits of consumerist pleasure-seeking, just try to have what many people call a 'good night out' without money.)

So, I would suggest that a virtue ethics approach to long-term conditions might in the first place want to put quite a lot of question marks against the sort of society that marginalizes and ignores the experiences, needs, values and virtues of those living with long-term conditions. And this extends far beyond simply trying to get those who experience those conditions to participate fully in the employed, monetary economy. It may be that there are assumptions about the meaning and fullness of life that extend far beyond employment, consumer choice and the elimination of all that disrupts the free flow of money round the globe. The norm of a human being fully alive should not be automatically assumed to be the obedient wage-slave who works hard for ends that are not quite clear and goods that do not quite satisfy. Insofar as people with long-term conditions are measured against that norm and disparaged because of it, they should resist on their own behalf and that of us all. (That is, of course, quite different from saying that people with long-term conditions should not have an understood and honoured place in the social and economic order.)

Perhaps people with long-term conditions and those who share their lives have something very valuable to teach the whole community, not only about the purposes, possibilities and limits of human living, but also about the virtues that are needed to cope with these. If we are all brought up to cultivate the virtues of unbridled competition and individual ambition within the market economy, when we can no longer participate fully in that economy, when we retire or acquire some long-term condition that is not susceptible to quick remedy, then we will not have the resources of character and person, the virtues and values, which will be required to live fully in those circumstances. The very things that may have made us successful bread-winners or career people, our detachment, our impatience, our determination to sort things out quickly, may actually be impediments to flourishing within our changed life circumstances. Having to deal with dependence, uncertainty, lack of autonomy, or lack of esteem deriving from role or money, may literally drive us mad or at least make us very depressed.

In a world where suffering, impairment and pain are feared, ignored and wherever possible eliminated or hidden, we are not well prepared for an experience which is increasingly likely to be part of the one life that we live here. So it is very much in our interests to learn to think about another set of values and virtues that might serve us well outside the conventional workplace. I have already spoken of the virtues of patience, fortitude, kindness, appreciation, restraint, courage, serenity and practical wisdom that I found in Donald. This was far from passive quiescence – Donald could be very sharp when the Council failed to deliver on its promises of support and equipment or carers were needlessly rushed and careless.

How is this practical wisdom and different set of values and virtues to be acquired? Many people with long-term conditions and those who work with them are very knowledgeable and interested about all aspects of their situation and may often share their experiences with others in a similar position. However, ordinary members of the public are never invited to think about the virtues required for living with and supporting people with long-term conditions unless they, or people close to them, acquire these conditions. Their education into new values and virtues is usually undertaken perforce rather than willingly. For some people who acquire long-term conditions, understandably, they never relinquish attachment to the old virtues and attitudes that served them so well in their former lives. They may then fail to maximize the potential in their new situation, looking on the world and their own situation with increasing resentment and anger. But the question for us all is, Is there anything that we could do as a society to ensure that we help people to think about the virtues and values that they might need in future situations different from the present?

Some help is now often offered to people approaching retirement. They are encouraged to think that they need to plan their exit from the workplace and think about their values and activities for the future. But as far as I know, there is no real education, except perhaps in the discipline of philosophy, for the general public in thinking about how to cope with long-term restriction, loss, marginalization, uncertainty and diminishment. We are just supposed to work it out for ourselves if we are unfortunate enough to find ourselves in that position if and when it happens. This seems a poor way both of sharing and valuing common human experience and also of preparing us for all the possibilities that life may throw at us.

I am not suggesting that all primary school children need systematically to contemplate mortality on a regular basis, or that we should encourage people to entertain visions of their own possible illnesses and disabilities all the time. But it does seem like a peculiar form of denial if we never think about who and what we are and how we are going to cope with situations at all until the need is thrust upon us. Death, diminishment and disease are a real part of life. Like any other situation in life like sex, bereavement and marital breakdown, it would surely be helpful if we could be helped to develop or even just think about some of the virtues that are appropriate to survival and flourishing in different situations. We might come to question the values of capitalist society generally and health care in particular, perhaps to the benefit of ourselves and our fellow citizens. We should work to live, not live to work. Our value and values should not be solely contingent on our participation in the material goodies of the market economy.

Without meaning to do so in any way, Donald, through his living fully with and through a long-term condition, taught me by example (and virtues are usually embodied in action, not just in words), that there are other ways of living and responding than I had realized. He showed me that in what I might think of as intolerable conditions it is still possible to grow and flourish, to find pleasure and potential in life. He was well-off and had had many chances in life, so he did not have to endure many of the hardships and injustices that blight the lives of others with long-term conditions at a very basic level. Thus, he was no-one special, but in his own way, certainly worthy of moral praise and emulation.

As I myself approach old age, I wonder how I and others like me might acquire the virtues that are needed to prosper in the midst of considerable problems, limitations and adversity. I am not thinking here about being grateful for small mercies or knowing your place, or thinking that there are other people worse off than you are, 'so you have to have a sense of humour, don't you?'. Nor am I talking about producing saints who have to repress their real frustrations and feelings to keep up an acceptable face. I am wondering about how we all might learn to acquire the flexibility and solidity of virtues and values that will enable us to endure the unwished for, undesired, diminishing, and depleting well enough to have lives that are of value to us and those around us. The need for this kind of practical virtue formation seems now to me to be urgent. But I am not sure that I see any real attempt to learn voluntarily from the experience of those people living with long-term conditions how to create a new sense of virtues and values amongst those who may need them in future.

One thing I am sure about, however. There is considerably more to a valued and valuable life than cultivating the virtues of being a good employee at the expense of all other relationships and values.

Summary

This chapter has followed the train of thought of an ethicist as he has struggled to answer the question: Are there ways that people can prepare themselves in case they develop a long-term condition in the future? Using 'virtue ethics' and the 'ethics of character' the chapter has used a personal story to illuminate and analyse the sort of societal changes that might be needed to come to terms with the growing number of people living with long-term conditions. Individuals also have their own unique ways of dealing with adversity, such as the diagnosis of a long-term condition. Perhaps we should all have lessons to learn how to cope better if and when a long-term condition eventually affects us?

Further reading

Campbell, C. (1987) *The Romantic Spirit and the Spirit of Modern Consumerism*. Oxford: Blackwell.

Giddens, A. (1991) *Modernity and Self-Identity*. Cambridge: Polity Press.

Giddens, A. (1992) *The Transformation of Intimacy*. Cambridge: Polity Press.

Lasch, C. (1991) *The Culture of Narcissism*. New York: W. W. Norton.

Nussbaum, M. (1994) *The Therapy of Desire: Theory and Practice in Hellenistic Ethics*. Princeton, NJ: Princeton University Press.

Ritzer, G. (2006) *McDonaldisation: The Reader*, 2nd edn. Thousand Oaks, CA: Pine Forge Press.

For more on virtue theory generally, its roots, and its contemporary revival and relevance see:

Crisp, R. and Slote, M. (eds) (1997) *Virtue Ethics*. Oxford: Oxford University Press.

Darwell, S. (ed.) (2003) *Virtue Ethics*. Oxford: Blackwell.

Pence, G. (1993) 'Virtue theory' in P. Singer (ed.), *A Companion to Ethics*. Oxford: Blackwell. pp. 249–58.

Swanton, C. (2003) *Virtue Ethics: A Pluralistic View*. Oxford: Oxford University Press.

References

Aristotle (2003) *The Nicomachean Ethics*. Oxford: Oxford University Press, abstracted in S. Darwall (ed.), *Virtue Ethics*. Oxford: Blackwell. pp. 25–35.

Campbell, C. (1987) *The Romantic Spirit and the Spirit of Modern Consumerism*. Oxford: Blackwell.

Darwell, S. (ed.) (2003) *Virtue Ethics*. Oxford: Blackwell.

Giddens, A. (1991) *Modernity and Self Identity*. Cambridge: Polity Press.

Giddens, A. (1992) *The Transformation of Intimacy*. Cambridge: Polity Press.

Kings Fund (2010) *Long-term Conditions* [Online]. Available at: http://www.kingsfund. org.uk/topics/longterm_conditions/ (accessed 30 October 2010).

Lasch, C. (1991) *The Culture of Narcissism*. New York: W.W. Norton.

Nussbaum, M. (1994) *The Therapy of Desire: Theory and Practice in Hellenistic Ethics*. Princeton, NJ: Princeton University Press.

Pence, G. (1993) 'Virtue theory' in P. Singer (ed.), *A Companion to Ethics*. Oxford: Blackwell. pp. 249–58.

Ritzer, G. (2006) *McDonaldisation: The Reader*, 2nd edn. Thousand Oaks, CA: Pine Forge Press.

Swanton, C. (2003) *Virtue Ethics: A Pluralistic View*. Oxford: Oxford University Press.

Index